EARL MINDELL'S SHAPING UP WITH VITAMINS

"A lively new ~~~~~~
—Los Angeles Times

"You'll want to add it to your library of bodybuilding lit."
—Muscle & Fitness

"Solid ideas on attaining fitness...[and] to troubleshoot health problems."
—Booklist

"Easy-to-digest...contagiously enthusiastic."
—Publishers Weekly

"With our obsession for physical fitness growing every day, it's a pleasure to find another book by Earl Mindell....It is impossible not to be caught up in the spirit of his ideas."
—Ocala Star-Banner

* * * * *

ABOUT THE AUTHOR

A highly respected member of the American Nutrition Society, the National Health Federation, and numerous other pharmaceutical and health organizations, Dr. Earl Mindell has been a pharmacist/nutritionist for over twenty years. He is the author of the multi-million copy international bestseller *Earl Mindell's Vitamin Bible*, a book recently cited in *Time* magazine as a reference book of celebrity weight trainer Dan Issacson. The writings of Earl L. Mindell, R.Ph., Ph.D., have brought him recognition as one of America's most trusted and sought-after authorities on health and dietary supplements.

Also by Earl Mindell

Earl Mindell's Vitamin Bible

Published by
WARNER BOOKS

EARL MINDELL'S SHAPING UP WITH VITAMINS

How the Right Foods and Nutrients Can Help Shape Up Your Body, Your Mind, and Your Sex Life

Earl Mindell

WARNER BOOKS

A Time Warner Company

WARNER BOOKS EDITION

Copyright © 1985 by Earl Mindell and Hester Mundis
All rights reserved.

Book design by H. Roberts Design

Warner Books, Inc.
1271 Avenue of the Americas
New York, N.Y. 10020

A Time Warner Company

Printed in the United States of America

This book was originally published in hardcover by Warner Books.
First Printed in Paperback: June, 1986

10 9 8

This book is dedicated to Gail,
Alanna, Evan, my parents and families,
my friends and associates,
and
to the health, happiness, and
lifetime fitness of people everywhere.

Contents

TIME OUT

TIME OUT

Acknowledgments

I wish to express my deep and lasting appreciation to my friends and associates who have assisted me in the preparation of this book, especially J. Kenney, Ph.D.; Linus Pauling, Ph.D.; Harold Segal, Ph.D.; Bernard Bubman, R.Ph.; Mel Rich, R.Ph.; Sal Messineo, R.Ph.; Arnold Fox, M.D.; Dennis Huddleson, M.D.; Stuart Fisher, M.D.; Robert Mendelson, M.D.; Gershon Lesser, M.D.; David Velkoff, M.D.; Rory Jaffee, M.D.; Donald Cruden, O.D.; Joel Strom, D.D.S.; Nathan Sperling, D.D.S.; Peter Mallory; and Hester Mundis.

I would also like to thank the Nutrition Foundation; the International College of Applied Nutrition; the American Medical Association; the New York Blood Center; the American Academy of Pediatrics; The American Dietetic Association; the National Academy of Sciences; the National Dairy Council; the Society for Nutrition Education; the United Fresh Fruit and Vegetable Association; the Albany College of Pharmacy; Betty Haskins; Lynn Harraton; Stephanie Marco; Susan Towlson; Ronald Borenstein; Laura Borenstein; and Richard Curtis, without whose professioal guidance and wise counsel a responsibility of this magnitude could not have been authoritatively discharged.

Preface

The vital connection between exercise, nutrition, and health has become one of the most important facts of life. This is not to put down the birds and bees, who have known it right along, since they work out daily, eat the right foods, and, to my knowledge, have never needed medical insurance. Nonetheless, facts of life are often confusing, and this latest is probably the most confusing of all.

Regrettably, the plethora of information now available on the subject is so overwhelming (and in many instances incredibly technical) that anyone trying to sort it out inevitably winds up more frustrated than informed. Because of this and my firm belief that everyone is entitled to optimal health, I felt that there should be a single book that could serve not only as an uncomplicated and comprehensive guide to all aspects of fitness but also as a convenient home reference for individual and changing needs—and I made up my mind to write it.

As a nutritionist and pharmacist, I learned long ago that the average person is a myth. No one vitamin or exercise regimen fits all, which is why I've designed this book so that it could be self-tailored as much as possible to suit individuals, not statistics.

I have avoided the use of age as a major separating factor since I've known sixty-year-olds in better shape than many thirty-year-olds and believe that maximizing health should be a goal for all time and not one limited by age.

Dividing the book into physical, emotional, and sexual shape-up categories, I have included in-depth nutritional and pharmaceutical information on aerobic and other workouts, energy, dieting, pregnancy, skin and body care, sexual function and dysfunction, depression, illness, drug abuse, and more.

Every section is numbered and cross-referenced, allowing you to quickly locate essential vitamin-drug-exercise interactions and cautions, specific health problems and considerations, natural remedies, fitness-potentiating (and debilitating) nutrients and medicines, as well as individualized supplement regimens developed for improving whatever fitness program you are on or whatever physical condition you are in.

Between chapters, I have inserted what I call a "Time Out," shape-up and nutrition facts that I believe are well worth thinking about—and acting on.

My recommendations in *all* instances are not meant to be prescriptive; they are offered only as suggestions, which should be discussed with your doctor. No book is or should be regarded as a substitute for professional care.

I have tried, though, to simplify and consolidate vast amounts of information to help provide everyone with enough knowledge to become a winner at health and fitness. And it is my sincerest desire for all readers of this book to do just that.

EARL L. MINDELL, R.Ph., Ph.D.

Beverly Hills, California
October, 1984

A Note to the Reader

The regimens throughout this book are recommendations, not prescriptions, and are not intended as medical advice. Before starting any new program, check with your physician or a nutritionally oriented doctor (see section 145), especially if you have a specific physical problem or are taking any medication.

EARL MINDELL'S SHAPING UP WITH VITAMINS

I.

Fitness for All

1. What Is Fitness?

Fitness, both emotional and physical, should be the goal of anyone who desires an energized and productive life. It is more than just the absence of disease. It's a feeling of all-over well-being that generates from good joint flexibility and muscular development, from healthy lung and heart stamina, and from the ability to exert reasonable stress on the body with positive invigorating results. It's a creative energy that allows us to greet each day and its tasks with confidence and enthusiasm.

> There are no diets or supplements that can take the place of exercise.

Inactivity is not conducive to fitness. Our hearts, lungs, muscles—in fact, all our organs—need exercise to keep them functioning at their best. There are no diets or supplements that can take the place of exercise, but when the right foods, supplements, and exercises are combined, the results are unbeatable!

2. Why You Need Energy

Energy is necessary for all bodily functions—even sleeping. Granted, more energy is needed for running a mile than for taking a nap, but it _is_ essential for both.

> The more active you are, the more energy you'll have.

The less active you are and the less energy you use, the less energy you'll have. Conserving energy, as far as your body is concerned, is an often misunderstood figure of speech.

Energy comes from the burning up of calories that we get from food, and oxygen is the fuel that's necessary to turn these calories into energy. In other words, no matter how well you eat, if your body's not receiving sufficient oxygen, you're not getting the benefits of energy.

The more active you are, the more stamina your oxygen-delivering systems will have—and the more active you can be.

3. How To Up Your Energy

- Exercise regularly.
- Avoid sugar-rich foods (a quick sugar high that elevates glucose levels is all too often followed by a period of low blood sugar and an even lower energy level).
- Don't become overweight (carrying around excess body fat drains energy).
- Keep your diet high in complex carbohydrates— vegetables, fruits, grain products—and low in sugars and fats.
- Increase your fiber intake.
- Avoid sleeping pills (they change sleeping patterns and usually leave you feeling not rested the following day).

- Drink 6–10 glasses of pure water daily, especially during warm weather (dehydration causes fatigue and can be dangerous).
- Keep away from stimulants (caffeine, amphetamines, etc.; those roller-coaster ups and downs take heavy energy tolls).
- Try meditation, yoga, or biofeedback to minimize daily stress, which can be a real energy depleter (see section 126).

4. Energizing Foods and Supplements

If you find that your "get-up-and-go" often doesn't do either, the following foods and supplements may be what you're missing.

ZINC

This important mineral governs the contractibility of muscles. A lack of it in your diet can increase fatigue and cause a susceptibility to infection and injury, as well as a slowdown of alertness. (Excessive sweating can cause a loss of as much as 3 mg. a day.)

Make sure your diet contains an ample variety of vegetables, whole-grain products, nonfat dry milk, brewer's yeast, wheat bran, wheat germ, pumpkin and sunflower seeds, fish, meat, and liver.

As a supplement, zinc is available in all good multivitamin and multimineral preparations. It can also be bought as zinc-sulfate or zinc-gluconate tablets in doses ranging from 15 to over 300 mg. (Both zinc sulfate and zinc gluconate seem to be equally effective, but zinc gluconate has been found to be more easily tolerated gastrointestinally. The chelated form is best.) Though zinc is virtually nontoxic—except when the food ingested has been stored in galvanized containers or there is an excessive intake—supplemental doses over 150 mg. daily could be harmful and are *not* recommended.

If you're a diabetic, a heavy drinker, or take large amounts of vitamin B_6, you need higher intakes of zinc. Keep in mind, too, that if you are adding zinc to your diet, you will increase your need for vitamin A. In fact, zinc works best in combination with vitamin A, calcium, and phosphorus.

VITAMIN A

This fat-soluble vitamin, which is stored in your body and generally doesn't need daily replenishment, promotes growth, strong bones, healthy skin; keeps the outer layers of tissues and organs healthy; and potentiates your needed zinc.

If your weekly diet includes ample amounts of liver, carrots, spinach, sweet potatoes, or cantaloupe, it's unlikely that you need an A supplement. But if you're often fatigued, you might have a vitamin A deficiency, in which case supplementation would be recommended.

Vitamin A supplements are available in two forms: one derived from natural fish-liver oil and the other water-dispersible. (Water-dispersible supplements are either acetate or palmitate and are recommended for anyone intolerant to oil, particularly acne sufferers.) The most common daily doses are 10,000 to 25,000 IU. Since vitamin A can build up in the system, I advise taking this vitamin only five days a week and then stopping for two. Toxicity can occur if more than 100,000 IU is taken daily for an extended period of time; doses of 18,500 IU daily can cause toxicity in infants. (Symptoms of toxicity include hair loss, nausea, vomiting, diarrhea, scaly skin, blurred vision, rashes, bone pain, headaches, and irregular menses, among others. If you notice any of these symptoms, discontinue use of supplement until you've consulted your doctor or a nutritionally oriented physician. [See section 145.]) Vitamin A works best with zinc, B complex, vitamins D and E, calcium, and phosphorus. It also helps vitamin C from oxidizing.

B-COMPLEX VITAMINS

These help release energy from the food we eat by converting carbohydrates into glucose and increasing our ability to fight fatigue. They also help form healthy red blood cells that deliver needed oxygen to the body.

The B-complex vitamins are Vitamin B_1 (thiamine), vitamin B_2 (riboflavin), vitamin B_3 (niacin), vitamin B_6 (pyridoxine), vitamin B_{12} (cyanocobalamin), vitamin B_{13} (orotic acid), pangamic acid, biotin, choline, folic acid, inositol, and PABA (para-aminobenzoic acid).

For optimal natural intake of B vitamins, your diet should include sufficient weekly amounts of liver, dried yeast, whole wheat, oatmeal, peanuts, vegetables, bran, fish, eggs, wheat germ, cantaloupe, cheese, root vegetables, brewer's yeast, whole brown rice, whole grains, pumpkin and sesame seeds, fruits, kidney, heart, raisins, unrefined molasses, cabbage, the white meat of poultry, avocados, dates, and bran. Milk, dairy products, and red muscle meat are also fine sources of B vitamins, but for some people milk and dairy products can cause mucous buildup and engender asthmatic-like reactions, which can hamper athletic performance. Additionally, these particular protein sources can deplete enzymes that are necessary to protect the body from injuries.

B-complex supplements are available in low-and high-potency dosages—and work best when vitamins B_1, B_2, and B_6 are in equal 50-mg. or 100-mg. balance. Because they are water-soluble vitamins, there is no known toxicity. (If taken in great excess, it's possible that symptoms such as tremors, edema, nervousness, rapid heartbeat, allergies, and neurological disturbances could develop.)

CAUTION: Anyone taking levodopa medication for Parkinson's disease should not take vitamin B_6.

If you're a heavy alcohol or coffee drinker, on the pill, under stress, or consume large amounts of refined carbohydrates, B-complex supplementation is recommended.

IRON

This mineral not only helps to prevent fatigue but also promotes resistance to disease, aids in growth, and is necessary for the proper metabolization of B vitamins.

The best natural sources of energizing iron that you can include in your diet are pork liver, beef kidney, heart and liver, farina, raw clams, dried peaches, red meat, egg yolks, oysters, nuts, beans, asparagus, and oatmeal.

As a supplement, the most assimilable form of iron is hydrolyzed protein chelate (organic iron that has been processed for fastest assimilation). This form is nonconstipating and easy on sensitive systems. Be aware that ferrous sulfate (inorganic iron), which is included in many vitamin and mineral supplements, can destroy vitamin E unless the two are taken eight hours apart. Supplements with inorganic iron—ferrous gluconate, ferrous fumerate, ferrous citrate, or ferrous peptonate—do not neutralize vitamin E, and are available in doses up to 320 mg., though daily doses over 75 mg. are rarely recommended. Toxicity is rare in healthy adults, but large doses or extended use of non-fortified vitamins can be hazardous for children.

Women are most likely to need iron supplementation—though most good multivitamin or mineral preparations will usually supply adequate amounts. Heavy coffee, tea, and cola consumers should be aware that these beverages can inhibit proper iron absorption.

CAUTION: Iron supplements should not be taken by anyone with sickle-cell anemia, hemochromatosis, or thalassemia. Pregnant women should not take iron or iron-fortified vitamin supplements without a doctor's prescription since iron poisoning has been found in children whose mothers have taken too much during pregnancy.

VITAMIN C

Though not an energizer by itself, vitamin C is essential for the formation of collagen, which is necessary for the growth and repair of body tissue, cells, blood vessels, and bones, and is a deterrent to energy-depleting stress and illness.

Because our bodies cannot synthesize vitamin C, it's important that your diet include adequate amounts of citrus fruits, berries, green and leafy vegetables, tomatoes, cauliflower, and potatoes.

As a supplement, vitamin C is available in just about every form a vitamin can take (pills, time-release tablets, syrups, powders, chewable wafers) and is available in tablet and capsule strengths up to 1,000 mg. (Powders go as high as 5,000 mg. per teaspoon.) The daily dosages usually range between 500 mg. and 4,000 mg. (4 grams). The best supplements are those that contain the complete vitamin C complex of bioflavonoids, hesperidin, and rutin, which are sometimes labeled citrus salts. (The only difference between natural or organic vitamin C and ordinary ascorbic acid is primarily the individual's ability to digest it.)

Because this is a water-soluble vitamin, toxicity is rare, though an excessive intake could cause oxalic-acid and uric-acid stone formation. (Taking magnesium, vitamin B_6, and a sufficient amount of water daily can usually prevent this.) High doses (over 10 g. daily) could cause unpleasant side effects— diarrhea, excess urination, skin rashes. Cutting back the dosage (which should be done slowly) will eliminate these side effects. If you are taking more than 750 mg. daily, I suggest taking a magnesium supplement also. This is an effective deterrent against kidney stones.

CAUTION: Vitamin C should not be used by cancer patients undergoing radiation or chemotherapy. Also, diabetics should be aware that vitamin C can alter results of urine tests for sugar, as well as other laboratory tests (particularly those to detect the presence of blood in stool). Before having any medical workups, inform your doctor if you are taking vitamin C.

If you exercise in any urban area, be aware that carbon monoxide destroys vitamin C, so up your intake accordingly. Also, if you've been taking aspirin to relieve the pain or inflammation of a workout injury, you should know that you're tripling the excretion rate of your vitamin C—and replenishment is in order.

CYTOCHROME C

This simple compound of amino acids and iron has become known as one of the foremost aerobic energy enhancers. It increases muscle performance, acts as a carrier of oxygen to the mitochondria (the cell powerhouse of skeletal muscle), and is an essential part of the metabolic process that makes prolonged exercise possible. In actively working muscles, the aerobic process of energy production is dependent on cytochromes. If this system becomes ineffective, the muscle cell metabolism switches to an alternate aerobic pathway that produces lactic acid. As the lactic acid builds, muscle fatigue ensues and thus reduces working endurance.

Cytochrome C is available in supplement form and is highly recommended for anyone who wants to get the best results from aerobic exercise.

INOSINE

Known as an antifatigue nutrient, inosine is found in meat, meat extracts, and sugar beets. A naturally occurring metabolic product that's readily utilized by the body, inosine increases the oxygen-carrying capacity of the blood, allowing more oxygen to be delivered to muscles and thereby reducing fatigue.

PROPOLIS

This energizer is a resinlike material found in leaf buds and the bark of many common trees. It is collected by bees, who use their enzymes to convert it into pollen.

Propolis is a rich source of minerals, B vitamins, and natural antibiotics. It has been shown to give athletes increased energy and staying power. It can also stimulate the thymus gland, enhance the body's immune system, and be used externally to heal bruises and blemishes.

As a supplement, it's available in tablet, granule,

and tincture form. (There are also creams available for external use.)

VITAMIN E

This is one of the most important nutrients for anyone who exercises, or wants to. It not only improves cardiovascular tone and circulation, which increases the amount of oxygen supplied to muscles and minimizes the accumulation of lactic acid that can cause muscle spasms, but it is also an excellent antioxidant. (When tissue oxygenation is increased by aerobic exercises, your need for antioxidants also increases.) Additionally, it can alleviate muscle cramps and charley horse.

Wheat germ oil is one of the best natural sources, particularly because it also contains octacosanol (see below). Other good dietary sources are soybeans, broccoli, brussels sprouts, leafy greens, whole wheat, whole-grain cereals, and eggs.

Vitamin E supplements are available in oil-base capsules, as well as water-dispersible dry tablets, and are supplied in strengths from 100 to 1,000 IU. Though it is virtually nontoxic, it is a fat-soluble vitamin that can be stored in the body. Excessive doses are not recommended without consultation with a nutritionally oriented doctor. (See section 145.)

City dwellers and people with chlorinated drinking water have a greater need for vitamin E, which enhances the effectiveness of vitamin A. When taken with 25 mcg. of selenium, vitamin E becomes more potent. Dosages should be increased (or decreased) gradually, and supplements should not be taken together with inorganic iron (ferrous sulfate), which can destroy vitamin E. (Take these at least eight hours apart.)

OCTACOSANOL

This is a remarkable energy sustainer that has been shown to dramatically increase athletic stamina. A natural food substance, which is present in very small amounts in vegetable oils, alfalfa leaves, wheat, wheat germ, and wheat germ oil, it has also been found to reduce heart stress and quicken reaction time.

Octacosanol is available as a supplement in tablet form (1,000–2,000 mcg.), but it may take four to six weeks before you notice measurable exercise benefits.

GINSENG

When your energy is low, ginseng can be just the pick-me-up you need. It's a stimulant, but *not* an excitant (in other words, there aren't high-low roller-coaster effects), and it's been found to increase physical endurance.

Ginseng also helps in the assimilation of vitamins and minerals.

As a supplement, it's available in capsule form, under names such as Siberian ginseng and Korean ginseng, in 500 mg. to 650 mg. (10 grain) doses, and can also be purchased as tea, liquid concentrate, or as ginseng root in a bottle.

Vitamin C has been said to neutralize part of ginseng's value, but there is no real evidence to support this. (If you take a vitamin C supplement, the time-release form makes any counteraction less likely.) To get the best energizing effects from ginseng, take it on an empty stomach.

AMINO ACIDS

Amino acids are the building blocks of protein (all proteins are made up of amino acids). They are used to synthesize other proteins—including muscle proteins—and are prime energy sources. They help break down fats for energy use, strengthen the body's connective tissue to prevent injury, improve mental alertness, quicken reflexes, elevate moods, and promote resistance to disease.

There are twenty-two known amino acids, eight of which are called *essential*. These, unlike the others, *cannot* be manufactured by the human body and *must* be obtained from food or supplements. (A ninth amino acid, histidine, is considered essential only for infants and children.)

The essential amino acids are isoleucine, leucine, lysine, methionine, phenylalanine, threonine, tryptophan, and valine. In order for the body to effectively use and synthesize protein, *all* the essential amino acids must be present and in the proper proportions. Even the temporary absence of a single essential amino acid can adversely affect protein synthesis and your energy benefits. In fact, whatever essential amino acid is low or missing will proportionately reduce the effectiveness of all the others.

Amino acid supplements are available in balanced formulas as well as in individual supplements. I'd recommend the former for general energy enhancement. And while taking an amino acid supplement, don't forget that you need enough vitamins B_6 and B_{12}, and niacin in your diet for proper metabolism.

5. Now That You Have Energy, Do You Need a Stress Test?

Not everyone needs a stress test before embarking on an exercise regimen, but if you're over forty years of age, or have a family history of heart disease, a full physical exam that includes a stress test is recommended.

Stress tests are *not* infallible!

Basically, a stress test is used to determine the heart's ability to send oxygen-containing blood to muscles as they are pushed to work harder. The test involves an ECG (electrocardiogram) and a monitoring of blood pressure and pulse rate, first when you're resting and then after performing a certain amount of exercise. (This is usually walking up and down a two-step stool or on a treadmill; sometimes riding a stationary bicycle.)

These tests are not infallible, though they can usually tell if you're a high risk for cardiovascular problems, which is essential for anyone considering strenuous sports and workouts to be aware of.

Equally important is recognizing that even if you do pass a stress test, it's unwise to rush headlong into any strenuous activity without having previously conditioned for it.

6. What You Should Know Before Choosing an Exercise

There are a wide variety of exercises available to everyone, but the best ones for you are those that meet *your* individual needs and capacities.

All exercises fall into one or more of four basic categories: isometric, isotonic, anaerobic, and aerobic. Understanding their dynamics—benefits and limitations—

will not only help you in selecting an exercise regimen but will also give you a pretty good idea of what to expect, in the way of fitness, from what you're doing.

7. Isometrics

Isometric exercises contract muscles without producing movement or demanding appreciable amounts of oxygen. In other words, they can increase skeletal muscle size and strength, but have few benefits to offer the heart, lungs, and circulatory system in general.

The key to isometrics is muscles working in equal measure against each other or some immovable object— for instance, trying to lift up the chair you're sitting on or pushing against opposite sides of a doorway. These types of exercises can be quite beneficial to bedridden patients by helping to prevent muscle atrophy or to regain limb strength. Unfortunately, they offer little to the average individual in search of general fitness.

8. Isotonics

Like isometrics, isotonic exercises work essentially on muscles, the difference being that isotonics contract muscles and *do* produce movement, while isometrics do not.

Isotonics are usually considered preferable to isometrics because the large muscles are at least being used rhythmically and repeatedly in some sort of continuous motion, as in weight lifting, for example. Nonetheless, cardiovascular benefits are minimal, and an exclusive isotonic exercise regimen is not advised for overall body conditioning.

9. Anaerobics

Anaerobic exercises are limited to short bursts of vigorous activity. They derive energy from the body's glycogen (sugar) reserves by processes requiring no oxygen (which, paradoxically, puts intense demands on existing oxygen supplies) and thereby restrict any exercise designed for duration.

Anaerobics are fine if your goals are all-out last-minute sprints because short, high-intensity-energy needs rely on a rapid breakdown of glycogen. Still, even though energy can be supplied rapidly by glycogen, it can't be easily stored in the body. Moreover, during anaerobic exercises, lactic acid (the muscle waste product that causes cramping and soreness) accumulates quickly and can injure muscles if not burned up or dissipated.

Any activity that you cut short because of lack of breath—either voluntarily (as in a preplanned bicycle sprint) or involuntarily (becoming winded after two laps across the pool) would be deemed anaerobic.

Anaerobics have their place in the training of athletes, but unless you're being coached by a professional, it's advisable not to demand more oxygen of your body than it's either been trained for or capable of giving.

10. Aerobics

The goal of these exercises is to increase your body's capacity to take in oxygen, and, by doing so, increase your stamina and endurance. These benefits (see section 15) are unquestionably amazing!

Effective aerobic exercise is based essentially on moderate intensity with long duration. (It's not what you do, but how long you do it that counts.) And when done correctly, they heap rewards on your entire body!

With aerobics, *time* is the essence. In other words, more benefits are gained by keeping an exercise's intensity low and manageable enough to continue working for the required length of time. (Twenty minutes, at least three times a week, is recommended for beginners.) And no matter what exercise you're doing, you must be able to sustain it for at least two minutes at a time without becoming winded. Monitoring your heart rate (see section 14) is a safe and simple way to evaluate how much you should or shouldn't be doing.

11. Mindell's Fitness Menu

The following are merely suggestions for achieving optimal fitness pleasurably. Every selection has aerobic benefits to offer, but the list is by no means meant to be all-inclusive.

As with any menu, the choices are up to you. You're limited only by your individual capacities and preferences.

WALKING

A four-star winner! As a leg- and buttock-toner, this should not be overlooked. If you're out of shape, start at 3 mph. For those who demand more aerobic benefits, work up to 5 mph. Additional details in sections 19 and 20.

CYCLING

If trim and firmer legs and buttocks are what you're craving, cycling can be the perfect bill of fare. For starters, 6–7 mph is enough. Work up speed gradually. For recommended supplements, see section 44.

ROPE JUMPING

A specialty of the house. Convenient, fun, and only ten minutes can provide the same aerobic benefits as thirty minutes of jogging.

ROLLER AND ICE SKATING

Forget about sighs over flabby thighs *if* you keep the skating continuous. No substitutions for the necessary time. See section 12 for how much you need.

AEROBIC DANCING

A gourmet total-toner—as long as you don't decide to sit too many out.

JOGGING

If the best in calves and thighs is what you're after, this all-around toner can certainly cut the mustard. It's recommended, though, to check sections 29 and 35 for cautions.

RUNNING

A more calorie-consuming version of jogging, with similar benefits *and cautions*.

SWIMMING

A less stressful special for anyone who's overweight, and an excellent exercise choice for anyone interested in shaping up the arms, chest, and tummy. There are no substitutions for duration (see section 12), so keep those air mattresses out of the pool.

RACQUETBALL

Recommended for fast, fun, full-bodied aerobic toning *if* you keep yourself in motion for at least half an hour.

ROWING

Whether you do it across a lake or on a machine in your home, half an hour nonstop is ideal body conditioning, and great for arm and leg tone-ups.

TENNIS

I'd suggest singles over doubles, mainly because they demand more movement on the court. For supplement accoutrements, see section 49.

SQUASH

An alternative to racquetball, with similar toning rewards, cautions, and supplements. See section 50.

CROSS-COUNTRY SKIING

A firming favorite for arms, buttocks, calves, and thighs that will serve any body benefits— providing you don't stop at every alpine lodge along the trail. Recommended supplements are in section 45.

VOLLEYBALL

A vitality-giving specialty that can tone you inside and out—provided you keep in motion for the recommended amount of time. See section 12.

YOGA

An Eastern *pièce de résistance*. It can relieve tension, elasticize the spine, tone flabby muscles, increase endurance for participation in more strenuous activities—and much, much more. See section 53.

12. How Much Exercise Do You Need?

To really make a difference in how you look and feel, you should exercise at least twenty to thirty minutes three (preferably five) times a week.

For developing and maintaining true aerobic fitness, the American College of Sports Medicine (ACSM) recommends fifteen to sixty minutes of continuous aerobic activity (high intensity for short duration or low intensity for long duration) three to five days a week, working at 60 to 90 percent of your aerobic capacity. (See section 13.)

13. Know Your Exercise Limits and Goals

In order to get maximal benefits from exercise, you should know when to safely push yourself to your physical limit—*without overexertion*. This means being able to put yourself in the right target zone.

Your target zone is somewhere between 70 and 85

percent of the maximum rate your heart can achieve. (Exercise that causes you to fall below this level is not producing sufficient beneficial effects. Exercise that causes you to exceed this level is too stressful and should be scaled down.)

14. Determining Your Target Heart Zone

To determine your target zone, subtract your age from 220 (the average maximum number of heartbeats per minute for a healthy, fit adult), then multiply by .70 to find the low end of your zone and by .85 to determine the high end. (See chart below.) Count your pulse beats for ten seconds and then multiply by six (or count for fifteen seconds and multiply by four). As your fitness increases, you might have to heighten the intensity of your exercises to keep your heart rate within the target zone.

TARGET HEART ZONE

	AVERAGE HEARTBEATS PER MINUTE		
AGE	MAXIMUM	LOW	HIGH
25	195	136	165
26	194	135	164
27	193	135	164
28	192	134	163
29	191	133	162
30	190	132	161
31	189	132	160
32	188	131	159
33	187	130	158
34	186	130	158
35	185	129	157
36	184	128	156

	AVERAGE HEARTBEATS PER MINUTE		
AGE	MAXIMUM	LOW	HIGH
37	183	128	155
38	182	127	154
39	181	126	153
40	180	125	152
41	179	125	152
42	178	124	151
43	177	123	150
44	176	123	149
45	175	122	148
46	174	121	147
47	173	121	147
48	172	120	146
49	171	119	145
50	170	118	144
51	169	118	143
52	168	117	142
53	167	116	141
54	166	116	141
55	165	115	140
56	164	114	139
57	163	114	138
58	162	113	137
59	161	112	136
60	160	111	135
61	159	111	135
62	158	110	134
63	157	109	133
64	156	109	132
65	155	108	131

Beginners should monitor their heart rate frequently during workouts. (It's best to take your pulse at the wrist as the neck pulse is usually more variable.)

- Keep in mind that these are approximate numbers. If you are in extremely good condition, your maximum heart rate will probably be higher than your age indicates; if you're a smoker, it will be lower.
- If you find yourself at the high end of your target zone, intersperse exercise with intervals of walking.
- If you are unable to easily carry on a conversation while exercising, you're probably working too hard.
- You can prevent unnecessary stress on your body by preceding and following workouts with less strenuous warm-up and cool-down exercises. (See sections 23 and 26.)
- If you resume exercising after having stopped for a week or more, begin again at a lower level.

15. What Exercise Can Do for You

A lot! And the list continues to grow daily!

- *Lower blood pressure* (Although blood pressure might rise initially, regular exercise will lower it. Even hypertensives who have failed at dieting have found they can improve their condition through exercise.)
- *Alleviate depression* (See sections 122–124.)
- *Ease chronic or frequent back pain* (Yoga and stretching exercises have produced remarkable results. See Section 53.)
- *Improve the immune system* (Regular exercise increases the number of white cells—which fight disease.)
- *Help relieve discomforts of premenstrual syndrome* (PMS) (See section 108.)
- *Aid in the treatment of eating disorders* (See section 67.)
- *Provide relief for rheumatoid arthritis.*
- *Help retard the development of atherosclerosis.*
- *Reduce the risk of heart attack.*

- *Lower cholesterol levels* (It also improves the blood's ability to dissolve clots.)
- *Help in the treatment of diabetes* (Improves glucose tolerance.)
- *Aid in weight control* (See sections 55 and 56.)
- *Reduce the risk of osteoporosis* (brittle bones) (See section 110.)
- *Increase energy.*
- *Promote healthier skin* (See section 88.)
- *Improve learning capacity.*
- *Aid in more effective metabolism of nutrients* (Especially protein, iron, the B vitamins, and vitamin C.)

16. Nutrients That Can Maximize Exercise Benefits

Exercise cannot provide optimal fitness without proper diet, and vice versa. Though many people are aware of this, most do not realize that for every exercise benefit there is a nutritional counterpart. Knowing the nutrients that can potentiate your exercise goals is like having an inside tip on a horse race or a stock offer, the only difference being that you always come out a winner. (For foods containing these nutrients, see section 36.)

EXERCISE BENEFIT	NUTRIENT ENHANCERS
Lower blood pressure	Vitamin E, niacin, calcium, chromium, phosphorus, potassium
Alleviate depression	Vitamin B_1, magnesium, molybdenum tryptophan, tyrosine, phenylalanine
Ease back pain	Vitamins A, C, E: SOD (super-oxide dismutase)

EXERCISE BENEFIT	NUTRIENT ENHANCERS
Improve immune system	Vitamins A, C, D, pantothenic acid, iron, sulphur
Relieve PMS discomfort	Vitamins B_6, C, E, calcium, magnesium, manganese, evening primrose oil, pantothenic acid, dong quai
Aid in treating eating disorder	Folic acid, chlorine, zinc, dimethyl glycine
Relieve rheumatoid arthritis	Vitamins D, E, phosphorus, selenium
Retard atherosclerosis	Chromium
Reduce heart attack risk	Vitamins B_1, E, F, calcium, phosphorus, vanadium
Lower cholesterol	Vitamins C, choline, vitamin F (unsaturated fatty acids), inositol, niacin, phosphorus, vitamin P (bioflavonoids), vanadium, zinc, lecithin
Help in diabetes treatment	Vitamin C, GTF chromium, potassium, zinc
Aid in weight control	Vitamin F (unsaturated fatty acids), evening primrose oil, potassium, spirulina
Reduce risk of osteoporosis	Vitamins C, D, calcium, magnesium

EXERCISE BENEFIT	NUTRIENT ENHANCERS
Increase energy	Vitamins A, B complex, C, D, folic acid, iron, manganese, phosphorus, iodine
Promote healthier skin	Vitamins A, A_2, B_6, D, E, F, biotin, folic acid, inositol, niacin, PABA, iron, sulphur
Improve learning capacity	Vitamin B_{12}, choline, manganese, potassium, zinc

NOTE: Choline should be taken with all B vitamins for optimal effectiveness.

17. The Great Nutrient-Exercise Misunderstanding

Practically everyone who is conscious of fitness knows that protein is one of the most important nutrients for the maintenance of good health, and is the major source of building muscles, blood, organs, tissues, and so on.

But protein is only one of the nutrients necessary for increased energy, proper food utilization, effective organ function, and cell growth. Carbohydrates, fats, minerals, vitamins, and water are equally essential.

> Heavy meat eaters can do themselves more harm than good.

Recent studies have shown that muscular activity does *not*, contrary to popular belief, excessively increase the need for protein (which, unfortunately, far too many people believe is simply another word for meat).

There are two types of protein—complete and incomplete.

Complete protein provides the proper balance of necessary amino acids and is found in foods of animal origin—meats, poultry, seafood, eggs, milk, and cheese.

Incomplete protein lacks essential amino acids and is not used efficiently when eaten alone. It's found in seeds, nuts, peas, grains, and beans. However, when it is combined with small amounts of animal-source protein, it becomes complete.

Mixing complete and incomplete proteins can give you better nutrition than either one alone. In fact, heavy meat eaters often do themselves more harm than good, since meat contains twenty-two times more phosphorus than calcium, and phosphorus needs calcium to be properly metabolized, resulting in the body being forced to use its own supply. Also, too much phosphorus can deplete the body of needed zinc and magnesium.

An active person's diet should be as well balanced as any other individual's, the difference being an increased energy (calorie) requirement. And this should come from proportionately greater amounts of complex carbohydrates in the diet than protein or fat.

But be aware that all carbohydrates are not the same!

Complex carbohydrates are unrefined. Their fibrous makeup allows the body to release and convert starches and sugars into a gradual, sustained flow of energy. They're found in such foods as whole grains, legumes, and fresh fruits and vegetables.

Simple carbohydrates are essentially junk food. They're sugar and starches that have been refined to the point of not only being unable to nourish your body, but to the point of depleting it of necessary nutrients.

18. How To Succeed at Exercise Without Really Trying

- Vary your exercise. Boredom breeds dropouts. Variety is not only the spice of life, it can keep you in the best of shape.

- Forget about perfection. Even if you think that you're a totally uncoordinated klutz, there are ways for you to shape up. Swimming—even the dog paddle—if done for twenty minutes is great for the circulation, and strengthens arm and leg muscles as well. And you don't need a partner to dance within the privacy of your home. (Half an hour of bouncing uninhibitedly to Michael Jackson can work wonders.)

- Mothers can combine quality time with exercise time. Kids love it. In fact, if you establish a routine, *they'll* make you stick to it. (If you keep in mind that what you're doing is fun and not a chore, you'll get better results working with junior than with Fonda.)

- Use stairs instead of escalators whenever possible.

- If you're an outdoor exerciser, keep a jump rope handy for rainy days. (Ten minutes equals half an hour's jog.)

- If you're limber and loose-jointed, you'll find that aerobic dancing, gymnastics, roller and/or ice skating can turn work into play. (To find out if you are limber, try joining your hands behind your back. If your fingers lock easily, you're loose-jointed. If your fingers don't lock easily, the above-mentioned activities could frustrate and discourage you. You'd be better off, and have more fun, cycling, running, hiking, or playing racquetball.)

- If you're small-framed, select exercises and sports where lightness gives you an advantage. For example, swimming, gymnastics, horseback riding, or running.

- If you're underweight, go for activities that are going to build up your strength and endurance *without* discouraging you. You could start with simple calisthenics or running. In fact, surprisingly enough, weight lifting (under supervision) might be just what you've been looking for.

- Just because you're underweight doesn't mean that exercise has to be work. Unless medically contraindicated, fat-burning exercises such as swimming, aerobic dancing, race-walking, cycling, and yoga can be amazingly beneficial and fun.

- When watching TV, sit cross-legged on the floor. You'll be exercising your ball-and-socket hip joints (which can help prevent osteoarthritis) and not even know it.

- How about walking to work? If it usually takes you 20–30 minutes by mass transportation, chances are you'll arrive faster and healthier by walking. (And you won't even realize that you're exercising!) If the distance is greater, get off the train or bus at a station that will still allow you a 20-minute walk to your job. For commuters who use cars, I recommend parking at least 15 minutes away from your office. The walks to and from your vehicle will make it more than worth your while—and could even save you money.

19. What You Should Know About Walking

It's the simplest, most underrated exercise around, and yet one of the best. Rapid walking, for instance, requires more steps per minute than running, and actually involves more muscular activity.

> Walking can decrease appetite and improve memory.

Walking redirects the blood flow away from the digestive tract and helps you lose weight by decreasing appetite. It stimulates your system and burns up those hard-to-reach fats instead of easily available sugar.

By starting at a slow pace and increasing speed over a period of months, walking has been shown to improve short-term memory as well as reasoning faculties—especially in persons over the age of fifty-five.

20. Getting into Step

As simple and natural as walking is, if you plan to employ it as exercise, you should familiarize yourself with the following guidelines:

- Gradually establish your walking time, distance, and speed.
- For beginners: Recommended speed 2–4 mph (approximately 60–120 steps per minute).
- *The Complete Book of Exercise Walking* by Gary D. Yanker (Contemporary Books) suggests building up from 15–45 minutes daily over a period of four to six weeks. (Fifteen-minute sessions should be done five times weekly; forty-five minute walks every other day.)
- After the beginner stage, your walks should last from 45 to 75 minutes (daily distance in the 3–4 mile range).
- When walking, keep your shoulders, ankles, and knees relaxed, feet pointed straight ahead, and your head aligned as best you can over your body. (For faster walking, bend arms at a 90-degree angle to conform with your quicker leg movements.)
- Your weight should always be slightly forward, over your front foot and ready for the next step.
- Walking shoes should have ample room for your toes, but still grip your heel to prevent rubbing.
- Socks that absorb perspiration well are advisable.
- If you develop irritations or red spots, cushion them with moleskin.
- To increase aerobic walking intensity without increas-

ing speed, use weight—a backpack, hand weights, weighted belt, etc.

- Do not continue any walking exercise if foot pain develops, unless you have consulted a physician or a podiatrist.

21. A Splash Course in Swimming Fitness

Swimming exercises virtually every muscle in the body, but before you take the plunge, it's important to warm up your joints and stretch your body properly. (See sections 23 and 24.)

> For older persons or for out-of-condition swimmers, the breaststroke is the best.

The director of swimming at the National Sports Center in England recommends beginning with small stretches at the side of the pool and then starting your swim with exaggerated movements to warm up your respiratory and circulatory systems.

The key is to build up to more difficult stretches—and *never strain*.

The Crawl	The best general training stroke. It builds basic stamina and is particularly good for the back.
The Butterfly	This is highly recommended for upper arm and chest development, but is usually too difficult for most occasional swimmers.
The Backstroke	Best for those who find putting their faces in the water difficult; allows for easier breathing because face is never submerged.

The Breaststroke   Gentler than other strokes and good for older persons or for anyone out of condition.

For supplements to help swimmers, see section 40.

22. Weather To Exercise—Or Not

Dr. E. C. Frederick, research director at the Nike Sports Research Laboratory in Exeter, New Hampshire, has found that the ideal temperature for strenuous exercise is 55 to 60 degrees Fahrenheit. Above or below this range, a substantial portion of body energy is used for heating or cooling, which reduces strength, stamina, and speed.

> The ideal temperature for strenuous exercise is 55–60 degrees Fahrenheit.

Exercising in the midday sun can cause the body to dangerously overheat. The hours before 10 A.M. and after 4 P.M. are the best for all outdoor workouts.

HUMIDITY

Humidity slows down the evaporation of perspiration, sabotaging the body's natural cooling process. Toweling off excess perspiration helps, but it's wiser to forgo outdoor activities if the temperature and humidity are above 70.

WIND

If the wind is against you, don't try for your usual goal. (Running against the wind will cost approximately 5 percent of your energy; cycling against it will cost you three times as much.) It is possible, though, to eliminate some of the energy drain by jogging, running, or cycling in single file with another person, trading off the lead at regular intervals.

POLLUTION

Humidity intensifies pollution, so if you're a city dweller, schedule your exercises on nonhumid days and when traffic is not at its peak.

SUPPLEMENTS FOR THE WEATHER-WISE

- Vitamin A, 10,000 IU, 1–3 times daily (5 days a week)
- Vitamin C, 1,000 mg., 1–3 times daily
- Vitamin E (Dry form), 400 IU, 1–3 times daily
- Selenium, 50 mcg. daily

23. The Low-down on Warm-ups

The most common mistake people make about warm-ups is thinking of them only as stretches. Stretching is definitely part of warming up, but not necessarily the first or even the most effective part.

Warming up doesn't mean just stretching.

Warming up means getting your blood moving, your muscles untensed, and your body ready to face a workout. Jogging—or even walking—in place beats stretching as a warm-up choice because it raises the temperature of *all* the body muscles and thus prepares them for whatever concentrated effort you're going to pursue.

The best time for stretches (see section 24), which are essential for flexibility and one of the best preventives against movement injuries, is immediately *after* warming up. Once muscles are warm, they will stretch more easily and tearing becomes less likely.

24. Stretching Dos and Don'ts

Stretching increases flexibility, which is vital for everyone—whether exercising or not. But with stretching, as with most things, there are right and wrong ways to go about it. Being unaware of the differences can not only deprive you of stretching's rewards but could also cause you injury and pain as well.

- DO stretch slowly, gradually increasing tension, and stop when the muscles feel tight.
- DON'T bounce or use jerking motions, or stretch to the point of pain.
- DO employ stretches that can be held for a minimum of 30 seconds. (If less, you won't get maximum benefit, and muscle fibers will tend not to relax completely, which is necessary if you intend to stretch farther without pain.)
- DON'T stretch an injured muscle. (Injured muscles don't regenerate.)
- DO warm up before you stretch. (Mild exercise or even a nice hot bath will do the trick.)
- DO repeat your stretching exercise after finishing your workout period. (Your body will be all warmed up, and you'll get increased flexibility benefit.)
- DON'T expect immediate results from stretching. It might take about 6 weeks for you to realize your increased flexibility.

25. Foods That Can Stretch Your Stretches

To reduce muscle spasms and leg cramps	Brewer's yeast, wheat bran, wheat germ, liver, kidney, heart, cantaloupe, cabbage, blackstrap molasses, milk, eggs, beef
To keep muscles functioning normally	Dried yeast, rice husks, whole wheat, oatmeal, peanuts, pork, most vegetables, bran, milk, shellfish, carrots, beef, artichokes, brains, kidney, dried beef
To improve balance	Liver, beef, pork, eggs, milk, cheese, kidney
To ease muscle pain	Nuts, fruits, brewer's yeast, beef liver, egg yolk, milk, kidney, unpolished rice
To lubricate joints	Citrus fruits, berries, green and leafy vegetables, tomatoes, cauliflower, potatoes, sweet potatoes
To help keep you limber	Kelp, olives
To aid in muscle reflexes	Nuts, green leafy vegetables, peas, beets, egg yolks, whole-grain cereals
To lessen arthritis pain	Fish, poultry, meat, whole grains, eggs, nuts, seeds
To keep youthful elasticity in tissues	Wheat germ, bran, tuna fish, onions, tomatoes, broccoli

26. What's So Hot About Cooling Down?

After strenuous exercise, a cooling-down period is essential. In fact, stopping abruptly can be dangerous, and for some people possibly fatal.

Strenuous exercise should be followed by a gradual cooling-down period to prevent a buildup of catecholamines, blood chemicals that are particularly dangerous to anyone whose heart is sensitive to stress.

The easiest way to cool down after exercise is simply to walk slowly for a while and then rest supine (on your back). See section 28 for playing it safe.

If you've recently suffered an injury, a cold compress or a cool soak *after* your cool-down period can be helpful.

27. How To Tell When Enough Is Too Much

If there's one thing I always try to emphasize, it's this: Exercise should make you feel *better*, not *worse!*

You may be pushing yourself too hard if after workouts...

- you become extremely tired;
- you become easily irritable;
- you have trouble sleeping, even though exhausted;
- your heart is still pounding and you have trouble catching your breath—long after you've stopped exercising.

If you notice *any* of these symptoms—slow down! Give your body time to adjust. If you sense that they are occurring regularly, *check with your doctor* to find out why you and your exercises are not compatible. (See sections 29 and 35 for cautions.)

WARNING: Discontinue *any* exercise immediately if you experience tightness or pain in the chest, severe breathlessness, lightheadedness, dizziness, loss of muscle control, or nausea. DO NOT RESUME EXERCISE WITHOUT CONSULTING A PHYSICIAN!

28. Play It Safe

Five minutes after exercising, check your pulse. Count the beats for ten seconds and then multiply by six (or count for fifteen seconds and multiply by four). If your pulse is over 120, you were pushing too hard. Wait five more minutes and check yourself again. Your pulse should be back below 100. If it isn't, ease up and pull back on your exercise regimen.

29. Know When Exercise Is a No-No

As wonderful as exercise is, there are times when it is indeed contraindicated and should not be undertaken without specific instructions from your doctor.

No matter how good you feel, you'll feel a lot better if you have a professional okay.

DO NOT EXERCISE WITHOUT MEDICAL SUPERVISION IF . . .

- You have any infectious disease, whether it's in an active, convalescent, or chronic stage;
- you have sugar diabetes controlled by insulin;
- you have recent—or a history of—internal bleeding;
- you have any sort of heart disease or unusual cardiovascular condition (irregular heartbeat, enlarged heart, angina pectoris, heart valve problems due to rheumatic fever, etc.);
- you have high blood pressure;
- you are excessively overweight;
- you suffer from any sort of kidney ailment;

- you are anemic;
- you have an acute or chronic lung disease or any condition that involves breathing difficulties;
- you have arthritis;
- you have any type of convulsive condition.

30. How To Handle Injury

The simplest way for any fitness buff to deal with injury is just to remember this acronym: RICE. It stands for Rest, Ice, Compression, and Elevation of the afflicted area.

> Keep active during the healing process.

It's advised that as an injury heals you should keep active, even though it might mean switching to a different type of exercise. Doctors no longer recommend that healthy individuals with an injury related to exercise remain immobile. Swimming, for example, has helped many a football-knee or tennis-elbow victim keep in shape, preventing injuries.

31. Be Wary of Over-the-counter (OTC) Pain Relievers

> Just because a drug is sold over the counter doesn't mean it's safe for you.

For pain or injury, aspirin (acetylsalicylic acid) has long been favored as the drug of choice. It is one of the three most popular OTC medications taken worldwide.

For exercise-related injuries, its benefits are numerous:

- It provides relief from muscular aches and pains.
- It reduces inflammation.
- It reduces fever.
- It provides relief for headaches, arthritis, bursitis, lumbago, sciatica, rheumatism, neuralgia, neuritis, toothaches, and more.

But few people realize that aspirin, like other common OTC pain-relievers such as Tylenol and Datril (acetaminophen), which reduce pain and fever but not inflammation, and Advil and Nuprin (ibuprofen), which work much the same as aspirin and can reduce inflammation, have potentially dangerous side effects.

Just because a drug is sold over the counter doesn't mean it's safe for you.

32. Side Effects and Drug Interactions of Popular Over-the-counter Pain Relievers

ASPIRIN

POSSIBLE SIDE EFFECTS:
- Stomach upset and gastrointestinal bleeding (which might cause or activate gastric or duodenal ulcers and delay healing).
- Produce occult bleeding.
- Triple the excretion of vitamin C (necessary for the growth and repair of body tissue cells, blood vessels, bones, and teeth).
- May produce such allergic reactions as hives, swelling, rashes, asthma attacks, wheezing, shortness of breath, and inflammation of the nasal mucous membrane.
- Prolong bleeding. (Because it is a blood thinner, it can

dangerously potentiate the effects of anticoagulants such as Coumadin, Panwarfin, and Panheprin.)
- Can cause dizziness and tinnitus (ringing in the ears).
- Can deplete your body of such needed nutrients as vitamins A, B complex, C, calcium, and potassium. (See section 36 for a quick reference list of foods containing these nutrients so that you can increase your intake of them.)

DRUG INTERACTIONS:
- Can react adversely with corticosteroids (drugs used to reduce inflammation, swelling, and relieve allergic reactions).
- Increase the hypoglycemic action of such antidiabetic medications as Orinase and Diabinese.
- Can block therapeutic effects of such antigout medications as Anturane and Benemid.
- Can interfere with proper therapeutic function of such antiepileptic medications as Depakene (valproic acid).
- May increase dangerously blood levels of methotrexate, a drug used to treat certain types of cancer and psoriasis.

CAUTION: A lot more products than you realize contain aspirin. The following list is not all-inclusive, so if aspirin is contraindicated for you, be sure to read your medicine labels carefully and check with your pharmacist to be sure.

COMMON MEDICATIONS CONTAINING ASPIRIN

Alka-Seltzer
Anacin
Ascodeen-3D
Ascriptin
Bayer Children's Cold
   Tablets
Bromo Seltzer

Buff-A-Comp
Buffadyne
Bufferin
Cama Inlay-Tabs
Cirin
Codasa
Congespirin

COMMON MEDICATIONS CONTAINING ASPIRIN

Cope
Coricidin
Darvon Compound
(though not Darvon,
Darvon-N, Darvocet-N,
and Darvocet)
Dolene Compound-65
(though not Dolene)
Duradyne DHC Tablets
Duragesic
Ecotrin
Empirin Compound
Emprazil
Excedrin
Fiorinol
Measurin
Midol

Monacet
Norgesic
Pabirin Buffered Tablets
Panalgesic
Percodan
Persistin
Progesic Compound-65
Rhinex
Rubaxisal
Salsprin
SK-65 *Compound* Capsules
(SK-65 Capsules are
aspirin-free)
Supac
Synalgos Capsules
Triaminicin
Vanquish

TYLENOL, DATRIL, AND OTHERS
(ACETAMINOPHEN)

POSSIBLE SIDE EFFECTS:
- Stomach upset
- Skin rash
- Hives
- Fever
- Injury to mucous membranes
- Reduced amounts of white blood cells and platelets in blood
- Liver damage (if taken in high doses)
- Anemia

DRUG INTERACTIONS:
- Can cause liver damage if you're a regular alcohol

drinker or on alcohol-containing medicines (which most cough syrups are).

ADVIL, NUPRIN, AND OTHERS (IBUPROFEN)

POSSIBLE SIDE EFFECTS:
- Intestinal bleeding
- Hives
- Asthma attacks
- Aggravate high blood pressure
- Can cause kidney failure in susceptible individuals (diabetics, the elderly)
- Dizziness and tinnitus (ringing in the ears)
- Bloated feeling, heartburn, constipation and/or diarrhea

DRUG INTERACTIONS:
- Can react adversely with alcohol, alcohol-containing medications, and aspirin
- Can cause kidney problems if taken with diuretics (water pills)

CAUTION: If you are allergic to aspirin (or other salicylates), do not take this medication without consulting your doctor. Virtually the same side effects, cautions, and drug interactions for aspirin can be applied to ibuprofen. Advil and Nuprin, which are now available OTC, are merely lower-dosage versions of the prescription drug Motrin, and are therefore not recommended for anyone with heart disease, high blood pressure, ulcers or other stomach problems, kidney problems, or for anyone who is currently taking anticoagulants (blood thinners) or any anti-inflammatory medicine.

If you are pregnant, do not take this—or any other medication—without consulting your doctor!

While taking this medication, be sure to increase

your intake of foods containing vitamins A, B complex, C, calcium, and potassium. (See section 36.)

33. Exercises and Drugs You Should Never Mix

Before engaging in any strenuous exercise that can raise body temperature, check with your physician— especially if you are taking any of the following medications:

- Antispasmodics or anticholinergics (drugs used to relieve intestinal cramping) containing atropine.
- Antihistamines (drugs for allergies). These can cause drowsiness, affect concentration, and possibly elevate blood pressure dangerously during exercise.
- Cogentin (benztropine mesylate).
- Inderal (propanalol).
- Historal, Plexonal, Urogesic (scopolamine, scopolamine hydrobromide).
- Thorazine, Promapar, Sonazine (chlorpromazine).
- Tricyclic antidepressants (amitriptyline, desipramine, imipramine, nortriptyline, and protriptyline).
- MAO inhibitors (usocarboxazid, phenelzine, tranylcypromine).
- Inhalation anesthetics (ether, haothane, nitrous oxide).
- Doriden (glutethimide).
- Amphetamines (central nervous system stimulants).
- Diuretics (drugs that increase urine secretion). These, combined with body water and salt lost through perspiration, can cause dehydration.
- Any OTC decongestant.
- Anticoagulants (blood thinners). These become *more* effective when the body temperature is raised.
- Digitalis (a small 2-degree rise in body temperature can make this heart medication 10–15 percent more toxic).

- Chloromycetin (chloramphenicol). This topical antibiotic ointment becomes less effective as temperature rises, and if you or the weather gets really hot, the medication can cause bacteria to grow faster.
- Caffeine. This is a vasoconstrictor and should be ingested sparingly during exercise, especially in hot weather.
- Antihypertensive (high blood pressure) medications can become more effective with heat and lower blood pressure too much.

34. Alternative Treatments from Nature's Pharmacy

Before rushing out and buying drugs for minor exercise injuries and discomforts, take a look at what nature's pharmacy has to offer.

Keep in mind that these suggestions are not prescriptive, nor are they meant to substitute for professional medical care.

ATHLETE'S FOOT

A hazard for anyone who frequents a public gym, this fungus infection responds very well to vitamin C powder or crystals applied directly to the affected area. Until the infection clears, it's best to keep your feet dry and out of shoes as much as possible.

BROKEN BONES

Naturally, you need a doctor to set a broken bone, but you can alleviate the frustration of waiting for it to mend by accelerating healing time with vitamins and minerals. My advice for getting back on your feet or into the swing is to increase your calcium and vitamin D intake. Daily supplements of calcium, 1,000–1,500 mg.; and vitamin D, 400–800 IU should do the trick.

For discomfort or pain during healing, try drinking chamomile, comfrey, or ginseng tea. These brews have been known to work wonders.

BRUISES

Bruises are bound to occur if you're active in sports, but taking a vitamin C complex, 1,000 mg. (with bioflavonoids, rutin, and hesperidin) three times daily will help prevent capillary fragility, as well as speed up the healing of those black-and-blue marks.

A poultice made from comfrey, or a compress, applied externally, using comfrey tea, will usually relieve any pain.

LEG PAINS

If you're prone to these, increase your calcium. I'd suggest a chelated calcium-and-magnesium tablet, choline 500 mg., vitamin B complex 100 mg., and a chelated multiple mineral, taken with breakfast and dinner. Also vitamin E (dry form) 400–1,000 IU, one to three times daily. (Many sufferers from charley horse have found vitamin E enormously helpful.)

MUSCLE SORENESS

For that ache-all-over feeling after a workout, or when specific muscles hurt from being pushed too hard, a vitamin E supplement (dry formula), 400–1,000 IU, taken one to three times daily and a chelated multiple mineral taken with breakfast and dinner can help.

SPRAINS

Keep RICE in mind—Rest, Immobilization, *Cold* compresses, and Elevation to minimize swelling. Sprains are injuries to ligaments and tendons surrounding joints, and generally occur when the joint is forced into motion beyond its range. Since the signs of sprains—pain intensified by motion, swelling, tenderness, and often discoloration—are similar to fractures, it's important to elevate and immobilize the afflicted area, apply cold compresses, and contact a doctor.

Do not apply heat for the first twenty-four to forty-eight hours. This can increase swelling and pain. After that, though, warm or comfortably hot compresses or soaks are suggested because these will promote circulation. (A poultice made from comfrey will also help.)

To speed healing, I'd recommend the following supplements:

- Vitamin E (dry form), 400 IU, 1–3 times daily
- Vitamin C complex, 1,000 mg., A.M. and P.M.
- High-potency multiple chelated mineral, A.M. and P.M.
- High-potency multiple vitamin with chelated minerals, A.M. and P.M.

TENDON AND TISSUE INJURIES

Tendons, which surround joints, are vulnerable to tears and injury when stressed in active sports, which is why it's important to fortify yourself with enough vitamin C to produce ample collagen (the body's intercellular cement). For healing as well as for preventing injuries, I'd recommend:

- Vitamin C complex, 1,000 mg., 1 to 3 times daily
- Calcium pantothenate (pantothenic acid, vitamin B_5), 100 mg., 1–3 times daily
- Vitamin B complex, 100 mg., 1–3 times daily
- Choline, 500 mg., A.M. and P.M.
- A chelated calcium-and-magnesium tablet, 3 times daily
- Vitamin D, 400 IU, daily
- High-potency multiple vitamin with chelated minerals, A.M. and P.M.

35. Exercise Cautions

- If an exercise hurts while you're doing it, you're doing it wrong. PAIN MEANS INJURY!
- If any postexercise soreness doesn't disappear within 24 hours, you're doing yourself more harm than good.
- Sitting incorrectly while using an upper-body Nautilus machine could cause an injury that might keep you off the machine for weeks.
- Never wait until you are thirsty to drink. In hot, dry weather, sweat can evaporate so rapidly that you might lose several pounds worth of water without feeling dehydrated, and excessive water loss can cause muscle cramping and spasms.
- Women who overexercise can develop secondary amenorrhea, a cessation of normal menstrual function. (This is usually corrected when training levels are reduced and fat levels—and body weight— are increased.)
- You are more likely to injure your back if you do sit-ups with your knees straight. Keeping your knees bent is best. (Doing sit-ups every other day allows muscles time to recover.)
- Don't bounce when reaching for your toes. This acti-

vates nerve receptors in leg and back tendons, which tighten muscles—and tight muscles are more likely to tear. (Unlock knees slightly and then touch toes without straining.)

- Taking diet pills containing amphetamines and doing strenuous exercise can be a lethal combination, especially in very hot weather.
- When a muscle shakes or trembles during exercise, it's a sign of its weakness and could cause injury. (Rest for a few minutes before resuming exercise.)
- Never exercise immediately after eating. This not only interferes with the absorption of nutrients but can also cause severe cramping and discomfort.
- Don't stop strenuous exercise abruptly. This can be dangerous—and possibly fatal—for certain individuals. Strenuous exercise should always be followed by a gradual cooling-down period. (See section 26.)
- Women who are used to wearing high-heeled shoes should be sure to stretch their Achilles tendon (joins calf muscle to heel bone) and hamstrings (tendons binding hollow of knees) before beginning exercise.
- Do not undertake exercise without specific direction from your physician, if you have any sort of heart condition.
- City dwellers should be aware that air pollution is hazardous to outdoor exercisers because carbon monoxide lessens muscle endurance by crowding out oxygen from red blood cells.
- If you experience bronchial spasms during workouts, consult a doctor before continuing with your regimen.
- Don't force stretches or use jerky movements. This can cause tearing and injury of muscles and tendons.
- Intense aerobics can stretch unprotected joints to the point of injury if you are thin, even if flabby.
- If you have back pain, don't exercise without consulting a doctor. Incorrect exercise can worsen a ruptured disc.

- Before going for speed in any exercise, practice all new movements in slow motion several times.
- Repeated movement against resistance while holding air in lungs can raise blood pressure dangerously. (Learn how to breathe properly, if you're planning to lift weights or to use resistance machines.)
- When adding more stress to your workouts, be sure to increase your warm-up and cool-down periods accordingly.
- Drinking alcohol and exercising don't mix.
- Smokers should lower the intensity of their workouts. Proper duration is important, and smokers tend to tire more easily than nonsmokers.
- Older persons should not exert themselves to the maximum.
- Jogging and other active exercise can cause unwanted sagging in large-breasted women. (A good support brassiere can prevent this.)
- Avoid swimming in very cold water. If cold water enters the ear, it can result in disorientation, nausea, and possibly cause drowning.
- While engaged in any sport, don't suck candy, chew gum or tobacco. If you're knocked unconscious, these can lodge in your throat.
- If you get a nosebleed, don't tilt your head back (this could cause a swallowing of blood and vomiting). Apply pressure to the bridge of your nose and tilt your head to the side.

36. A Quick Vitamin, Mineral, and Amino Acid Reference List

VITAMIN	BEST NATURAL SOURCES
Vitamin A	Fish-liver oil, liver, carrots, green and yellow vegetables, eggs, milk and dairy products, margarine, yellow fruits

VITAMIN	BEST NATURAL SOURCES
Vitamin B_1 (thiamine)	Dried yeast, rice husks, whole wheat, oatmeal, peanuts, pork, most vegetables, bran, milk
Vitamin B_2 (riboflavin)	Milk, liver, kidney, yeast, cheese, leafy green vegetables, fish, eggs
Vitamin B_6 (pyridoxine)	Brewer's yeast, wheat bran, wheat germ, liver, kidney, heart, cantaloupe, cabbage, blackstrap molasses, milk, eggs, beef
Vitamin B_{12} (cobalamin)	Liver, beef, pork, eggs, milk, cheese, kidney
Vitamin B_{13} (orotic acid)	Root vegetables, whey, the liquid portion of soured or curdled milk
Vitamin B_{15} (pangamic acid)	Brewer's yeast, whole brown rice, whole grains, pumpkin seeds, sesame seeds
Vitamin B_{17} (laetrile)	A small amount of laetrile is found in the whole kernels of apricots, apples, cherries, peaches, plums, and nectarines
Biotin (coenzyme R or vitamin H)	Nuts, fruits, brewer's yeast, beef liver, egg yolk, milk, kidney, unpolished rice
Vitamin C (ascorbic acid)	Citrus fruits, berries, green and leafy vegetables, tomatoes, cauliflower, potatoes, sweet potatoes

VITAMIN	BEST NATURAL SOURCES
Calcium pantothenate (pantothenic acid, panthenol, vitamin B₅)	Meat, whole grains, wheat germ, bran, kidney, liver, heart, green leafy vegetables, brewer's yeast, nuts, chicken, crude molasses
Choline	Egg yolk, brain, heart, green leafy vegetables, yeast, liver, wheat germ (and, in small amounts, in lecithin)
Vitamin D (calciferol, viosterol, ergosterol)	Fish-liver oils, sardines, herring, salmon, tuna, milk and dairy products
Vitamin E (tocopherol)	Wheat germ, soybeans, vegetable oils, broccoli, brussels sprouts, leafy greens, spinach, enriched flour, whole wheat, whole-grain cerèals, eggs
Vitamin F (unsaturated fatty acids—linoleic, linolenic, and arachidonic)	Vegetable oils—wheat germ, linseed, sunflower, safflower, soybean, and peanut—peanuts, sunflower seeds, walnuts, pecans, almonds, avocados
Folic acid (folacin)	Deep green leafy vegetables, carrots, tortula yeast, liver, egg yolk, cantaloupe, apricots, pumpkins, avocados, beans, whole wheat and dark rye flour
Inositol	Liver, brewer's yeast, dried lima beans, beef brains and heart, cantaloupe, grapefruit,

VITAMIN	BEST NATURAL SOURCES
	raisins, wheat germ, unrefined molasses, peanuts, cabbage
Vitamin K (menadione)	Yogurt, alfalfa, egg yolk, safflower oil, soybean oil, fish-liver oils, kelp, leafy green vegetables
Niacin (nicotinic acid, niacinamide, nicotinamide)	Liver, lean meat, whole wheat products, brewer's yeast, kidney, wheat germ, fish, eggs, roasted peanuts, the white meat of poultry, avocados, dates, figs, prunes
Vitamin P (C complex, citrus bioflavonoids, rutin, hesperidin)	The white skin and segment part of citrus fruit—lemons, oranges, grapefruit; also in apricots, buckwheat, black-berries, cherries, and rose hips
PABA (para-amino-benzoic acid)	Liver, brewer's yeast, kidney, whole grains, rice, bran, wheat germ, and molasses

MINERAL	BEST NATURAL SOURCES
Calcium	Milk and milk products, all cheeses, soybeans, sardines, salmon, peanuts, walnuts, sunflower seeds, dried beans, green vegetables
Chlorine	Table salt, kelp, olives
Chromium	Meat, shellfish, chicken, corn oil. clams, brewer's yeast
Cobalt	Milk, kidney, liver, meat, oysters, clams

MINERAL	BEST NATURAL SOURCES
Copper	Dried beans, peas, whole wheat, prunes, calf and beef liver, shrimp and most seafood
Fluorine	Seafoods and gelatin
Iodine (iodide)	Kelp, vegetables grown in iodine-rich soil, onions, all seafood
Iron	Pork liver; beef kidney, heart, and liver; farina; raw clams; dried peaches; red meat; egg yolk; oysters; nuts; beans; asparagus; molasses; oatmeal
Magnesium	Figs, lemons, grapefruit, yellow corn, almonds, nuts, seeds, dark green vegetables, apples
Manganese	Nuts, green leafy vegetables, peas, beets, egg yolk, whole grain cereals
Molybdenum	Dark green leafy vegetables, whole grains, legumes
Phosphorus	Fish, poultry, meat, whole grains, eggs, nuts, seeds
Potassium	Citrus fruits, watercress, all green leafy vegetables, mint leaves, sunflower seeds, bananas, potatoes
Selenium	Wheat germ, bran, tuna fish, onions, tomatoes, broccoli

MINERAL	BEST NATURAL SOURCES
Sodium	Salt, shellfish, carrots, beets, artichokes, dried beef, brains, kidney, bacon
Sulfur	Lean beef, dried beans, fish, eggs, cabbage
Vanadium	Fish
Water	Drinking water, juices, fruits and vegetables
Zinc	Round steak, lamb chops, pork loin, wheat germ, brewer's yeast, pumpkin seeds, eggs, nonfat dry milk, ground mustard

AMINO ACID	BEST NATURAL SOURCES
Tryptophan	Cottage cheese, milk, turkey, bananas, meat, dried dates, peanuts, all protein-rich foods
Phenylalanine	Soy products, bread stuffing, cottage cheese, dry skim milk, almonds, peanuts, lima beans, pumpkin seeds, sesame seeds, all protein-rich foods
Lysine	Fish, milk, lima beans, meat, cheese, yeast, eggs, soy products, all protein-rich foods
Arginine	Nuts, popcorn, carob, gelatin desserts, chocolate, brown rice, oatmeal, raisins, sunflower and sesame seeds, whole wheat bread, all protein-rich foods

37. Any Questions About Chapter I?

Is it really true that you have to wait an hour after eating to swim?

It's best to wait even longer. Olympic athletes wait two and sometimes three hours. The length of time depends on your age and the temperature of the water. The younger you are, the shorter time you have to wait; but the colder the water, the longer you *should* wait. It's preferable with all exercise to stick to the hour-after-eating rule. Any time before that can interfere with the proper absorption of nutrients.

I've just gotten into running, and I'd like a little advice about diet. My brother (who's been running for three years) says that I should fill up on carbohydrates if I want real energy. Are these better than protein?

No one nutrient is "better" than another; they're all necessary. Carbohydrates and fats can be easily burned for energy, but without protein the body won't produce hormones that are necessary for energy production. Carbohydrate loading, which many athletes do before races, is often misunderstood. (See section 17.) There are good and bad carbohydrates, and consuming large amounts of sugars and starches—essentially junk foods—is not the way to fitness. In fact, refined carbohydrates such as these can cause water retention in muscles, interfering with contraction. And the quick burst of energy provided by sugary foods can, in the long run, result in nausea, cramping, and dizziness. (Refined carbohydrates can also raise cholesterol and triglyceride levels, undermining cardiovascular benefits that should rightfully be yours.) My advice is to simply vary your diet, favor complex carbohydrates over fats and protein for calories, cover all your nutrient bases, and wait at least three hours after eating before running to prevent your energy from being diverted to your digestive system.

I recently injured my ankle while skiing, and several friends recommended DMSO for rapid healing. I seem to recall reading, though, that this stuff has a lot of negative aspects. Could you tell me what they are, and what your advice is about using it?

Personally, I'm not in favor of DMSO (dimethyl sulfoxide), which is essentially a by-product of the paper industry that has, among other things, been used as an antifreeze. In the early 1960s, it was found to be a good anti-inflammatory drug that could be applied topically. But the Food and Drug Administration (FDA) discovered that it could rapidly enter the bloodstream and cause a loss of vision, nausea, skin rashes, and other unpleasant side effects.

I'm not always in complete agreement with the FDA, but as a pharmacist I do share its concern about DMSO's unknown purity and quality.

The drug has been approved for veterinary use, but as far as humans are concerned, it's approved only for treatment of a rare bladder condition known as interstitial cystitis. Formerly an under-the-counter drug that could be purchased only as a degreaser or as an art supply through the mail, DMSO is now available in health food stores. Used topically, it penetrates the skin and goes directly to the afflicted area. This may help reduce swelling and inflammation, but it also allows suspect or dangerous impurities from polluted air that settle on the skin to be carried into the bloodstream.

Until all the facts are in, I'd steer clear of it—and advise you to do likewise.

Aside from their unethical use in competitive sports, are steroids bad for you?

Sports medicine specialist Dr. Bernard Friedlander of Santa Monica, California, is convinced that prolonged use has definite harmful effects; pursuant to my own research, I have to agree.

Steroids produce a definite strain on the liver, and Dr. Friedlander's studies have also shown that they can cause damage to the kidneys and heart. Females have been found to develop deeper voices, larger muscles, and increased facial hair. On the other hand, men taking steroids often become prone to impotency.

Perhaps the biggest danger of steroids for those concerned with exercise, fitness—even competitive sports—is that they experience a deceptive sense of energy and can severely overstrain and injure their bodies.

I overheard a running friend of mine talking about the importance of orthotics. What are these? And how necessary are they?

Orthotics are usually used to guide the movement of the foot as it bears weight during walking or running exercise. They are made from cast impressions of the feet and are designed so they can be transferred to whatever shoes you are wearing. (Weight-bearing x-rays of the feet and a complete examination of your walking movements must be made for proper orthotics.) They're relatively expensive, but they can help keep the body in balance, prevent unnecessary foot injuries, and though I don't feel that they're necessary for all runners, they have proved beneficial to many professionals.

TIME OUT

Life's Essential Ingredient

The body can live weeks without food, days without
water, but just a few minutes without oxygen. The
role of exercise in increasing the body's ability to
take in and make use of oxygen is a critical one.

The President's Council on Physical Fitness

Think about it . . .

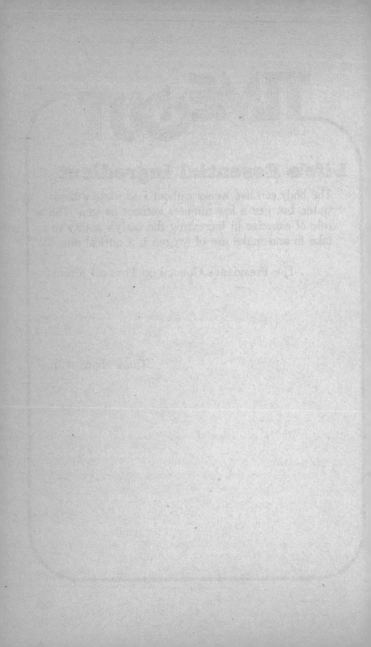

II.

Personally Yours

38. Your Special Vitamin Shape-up

All exercises make different demands on the body, and the body requires many different nutrients to meet these demands. In the following sections, I have outlined a number of personalized regimens for a variety of specialized exercise needs. I'd advise looking all of them over so if you discover that you fit into more than one category, you can adjust the combined regimens to avoid double-dosing and merely add the necessary additional vitamins.

Before starting any regimen, check "Cautions" (section 35) and with a nutritionally oriented doctor (section 145). *Please keep in mind that the regimens in this book are not prescriptive nor are they intended as medical advice.*

You will notice that in many cases I advise what I call an MVP, a Mindell Vitamin Program (which can make you an MVP—a Most Valuable Player in the fitness game). This basic vitamin trio is my foundation for nutritional health.

MINDELL VITAMIN PROGRAM (MVP)

* High-potency multiple vitamin with chelated minerals (time release preferred)
* Vitamin C, 1,000 mg. with bioflavonoids, rutin, hesperidin, and rose hips
* High-potency chelated multiple minerals

39. Runners

During the first fifteen to twenty minutes of running, almost only glucose is burned up. The body then comes in with fats (lipids) for energy. (In utilizing lipids for energy, a compound called acetyl-coenzyme-A is formed.) If there are only animal fats present, the compound forms slowly, and energy is insufficient (cut down your red meat intake). If, on the other hand, polyunsaturates are present, the compound forms quickly.

Increase your intake of polyunsaturates—seeds, nuts, whole grains, and antioxidants such as vitamins A, C, E, and selenium—to avoid free radical reactions.

SUGGESTED SUPPLEMENT PROGRAM

* Multiple vitamin with chelated minerals, 1–3 times daily
* Vitamin C complex, 1,000 mg., 1–3 times daily
* Stress B complex with zinc, 1–3 times daily

- Vitamin E (dry form), 400 IU, A.M. and P.M.
- Chelated multiple mineral tablet, 1 daily
- Cytochrome-C, inosine, and octacosanol, 1–3 times daily

40. Swimmers

If you take the plunge regularly, you're giving your entire body a fine all-over workout (See section 21.) But if you want to extend your energy, keep your muscles fortified and your skin from drying up, the following regimen is recommended.

SUGGESTED SUPPLEMENT PROGRAM

- MVP, A.M. and P.M.
- Stress B complex with zinc, 1–3 times daily
- Vitamin E (dry form), 200–400 IU, A.M. and P.M. (Aloe vera oil applied topically will help remoisturize water-whipped skin.)
- Cysteine, 1 g. daily (taken between meals with water— no protein)
- Cytochrome-C, inosine, and octacosanol, 1–3 times daily
- Vitamin C, 1 g. daily (in addition to MVP)

41. Fonda-philes

Jane Fonda's workout program offers multiple aerobic benefits, but as you progress to higher levels, more demands will be made on your body. Preparing for them now will make the difficult seem easier later on.

SUGGESTED SUPPLEMENT PROGRAM

- MVP, A.M. and P.M.
- Vitamin E, 200–400 IU, 1–3 times daily
- Lecithin capsules, 1–3 daily
- Extra chelated calcium, 500 mg. (to prevent muscle fatigue)
- Cytochrome-C, inosine, and octacosanol, 1,000 mcg., 1–3 times daily

42. Athletes

Instead of large amounts of protein, fortify yourself with complex carbohydrates.

The nutritional needs of athletes are more demanding than those of ordinary fitness-seekers. The prime nutritional requirement for performance is energy, and high-energy foods—as opposed to "quick-energy" foods—are what should be eaten. What you want as an athlete is more complex carbohydrates than protein or fat. (In fact, decreasing your intake of protein and fat and increasing complex carbohydrates boost athletic performance.)

After a grueling workout, what you need is not—as formerly thought—large amounts of protein. Moderate, even low, amounts of protein suffice, as long as you fortify yourself with an adequate supply of complex carbohydrates. These actually fuel the body, enabling dietary protein to be used more effectively.

Muscular pharmacologist Dr. David Lamb of Purdue University feels that 60 to 70 percent of an athlete's diet should be carbohydrates because they convert rapidly to glycogen, which is needed to regenerate the compound ATP (adenosine triphosphate) that initiates muscles to contract.

Avoid excess amounts of glucose, sugar, honey, or hard candy, which tend to draw fluid into the gastrointestinal tract and can promote dehydration problems in endurance performance. A thirst-quenching drink of tart fruit juice would be your best bet for a quick-energy beverage.

SUGGESTED SUPPLEMENT PROGRAM

- MVP
- Stress B complex
- Vitamin E (dry form), 400–1,000 IU
  All with breakfast, lunch, and dinner
- Cytochrome-C, inosine, and octacosanol, 1,000 mcg., 1–3 times daily

If you are in active training, you might add protein powder (which is low in fat) to your fruit juice. During this period, you would be well advised to use it as your main source of protein.

The night before your game or race, I'd suggest eating whole-grain pasta or bread, and drinking an unsalted vegetable juice, especially tomato, because it's a great source of potassium. On the morning of the event, complex carbohydrates are what you want. Be sure, though, that these products do not contain excess sugar, honey, molasses, corn or maple syrups.

43. Nautilus Buffs

Working mainly on the principles of isotonics and anaerobics, these machines have been designed to build all your muscles up to their maximum potential. Slow and steady sets the pace, and being nutritionally fortified helps you reach your individual goals faster. Increasing your intake of whole grains, brown rice, beans and apples, and other fiber-rich foods (see section 59) is advised.

SUGGESTED SUPPLEMENT PROGRAM

- MVP, with breakfast and dinner
- Vitamin E (dry form), 400 IU, twice daily
- Cytochrome-C, inosine, and octacosanol, 1,000 mcg., 1–3 times daily

44. Cyclists

Bicycling, whether indoor and stationary or outdoor and challenging, is excellent for aerobic conditioning, weight reduction, and general body-toning. (You can burn up nearly 400 calories in an hour if you go ten miles in that time.)

To avoid stress on the lower back, be sure that the bicycle you're using is fitted to your body. (Frequent backaches are often an indication that seat height or handlebars need adjustment.) Knee strain, which is quite common, can be prevented by raising the seat to a height that allows your leg full extension when your heel is on the pedal and the pedal is at the bottom of the cycle.

Other tips you might want to keep in mind:

- Changing your hand position on the handlebars frequently helps prevent aching arm muscles and finger numbness. (If upper-torso muscle aches are frequent, you might need to decrease the distance between the handlebars and saddle.)

- To prevent a sore bottom, try slipping a padded cover over the saddle.
- Biking can shorten muscles in the back of legs, so do warm-ups and stretches carefully before and after cycling. On chilly or damp days, keep your knees covered.

SUGGESTED SUPPLEMENT PROGRAM

- MVP, with breakfast and dinner
- Chelated calcium, 750 mg., with breakfast and dinner
- Vitamin E (dry form), 400–1,000 IU, 1–3 times daily

45. Skiers

Whether downhill or cross-country, skiing is a cold weather sport that requires the right clothes, foods, warm-ups, and cool-downs to give you fitness and fun rewards.

In freezing temperatures, the circulation in your hands and feet slows down because the body needs more blood to warm vital organs. (Doubling up on socks or gloves helps eliminate moisture and holds in heat.) Always wear clothing that's nonrestricting (avoid rubberized nonbreathing fabrics) and keep in motion as much as possible. (If there's a long line for the lift, walk in place while waiting; on the lift, unbuckle your boots to increase circulation.) And be sure to keep your head covered. It might only be one-eighth of your body, but uncovered it can result in a 95 percent body heat loss.

Dr. Bruce Craig, associate director of graduate studies at the Human Performance Lab at Ball State University in Indiana, recommends caution when working out in cold weather. (Warm-ups such as jogging in place and stretching should be done before going outside.) A face mask is advised, especially if you're not in top condition. Breathing freezing air rapidly through the mouth can be an unhealthy stimulus to the heart.

> Eat for heat. As the body metabolizes food, we feel warmer.

As the body metabolizes food, we feel warmer. But, according to Dr. Maria Simonson, director of the Health, Weight and Stress Program at Johns Hopkins University, you don't have to get fat to stay warm. Complex carbohydrates are the best foods for energy in any season, but you don't have to overdo them just because it's cold outside. For instance, Dr. Simonson recommends substituting a potato or a half-cup of pasta for a calorie-equivalent fruit. Complex carbohydrates have staying power, and by remaining in your stomach longer, they'll provide extended warmth. (See section 17.)

SUGGESTED SUPPLEMENT PROGRAM

- MVP, 1–3 times daily
- Niacin, 50–100 mg., 1–3 times daily
- Vitamin E (dry form), 200–400 IU, 1–3 times daily
- Chelated calcium, 750 mg., A.M. and P.M.
- Liquids (water, herb teas), 6–10 glasses daily (to prevent dehydration while exercising at high altitudes where there's less moisture.)

CAUTION: Avoid coffee, cocoa, and tea, which can act as diuretics.

46. Walkers

Walking is one of the best and easiest-to-master forays into aerobics. (See section 19.) It offers numerous benefits, requires minimum skill, and by simply doing it on a regular basis, you can tone up your entire body—inside and out. Nonetheless, you can maximize your fitness rewards by increasing the endurance-providing complex carbohydrates in your diet, such as whole-grain products, brown rice, vegetables, fresh fruit and vegetable juices; decreasing endurance depleters such as refined sugars, carbonated soft drinks, and junk foods; and using the following supplements.

SUGGESTED SUPPLEMENT PROGRAM

- MVP, 1–3 times daily
- Vitamin E (dry form), 200–400 IU, 1–3 times daily
- Chelated calcium, 750 mg., A.M. and P.M.
- Cytochrome-C, inosine, and octacosanol, 1,000 mcg., 1–3 times daily

47. Joggers

The nutritional needs of joggers are essentially the same as those for runners. (See section 39.) Polyunsaturates, whole grains, and antioxidants, such as vitamins A, C, E, and selenium, which help prevent free radical reactions, are important—especially if you're jogging in an urban area. (Foods you should include in your weekly diet are wheat germ, bran, broccoli, salmon, carrots, green and yellow vegetables, potatoes, and citrus fruits.)

Remember that with jogging, muscles are less subject to sprains, pulls, and tears if they're properly warmed up. (See section 23.) Cool-downs and stretches afterward (see sections 24 and 26) are also important because jogging can tighten tissues along the back of your body.

SUGGESTED SUPPLEMENT PROGRAM

- MVP, A.M. and P.M.
- Stress B complex with zinc, 1–3 times daily
- Vitamin E (dry form), 200–400 IU, 1–3 times daily
- Cytochrome-C, inosine, and octacosanol, 1,000 mcg., 1–3 times daily

48. Golfers

As much as you enjoy it, golfing often takes a lot more out of you than it gives. Its aerobic benefits come mostly from brisk walking across the course or from practicing your swing for an extended period of time at a driving range. Otherwise, it's a sport that does more for your ego than for your body. In fact, the stress and tension of the game can use up your B vitamins at a rapid clip. I can't say that supplements will get you down into the seventies, but they will help you stay energetic throughout the game—and could even put that extra zip in your swing that you've been trying for.

SUGGESTED SUPPLEMENT PROGRAM

- MVP, A.M. and P.M.
- Stress B complex with zinc, 1–3 times daily

49. Tennis Players

This is one of those sports that can keep you looking good while leaving you a nutritional mess. Dr. Robert Haas, who is tennis champ Martina Navratilova's personal nutritionist and the author of *Eat To Win* (Rawson Associates), recommends a diet that is low in fats and proteins (which if eaten in excess can actually drain energy) but high in complex carbohydrates—a clean-burning fuel that your body can quickly convert to energy (oatmeal, brown rice, lentils, and apples are good staples).

Far too many tennis players skip meals or eat only protein—both bad habits. A good serve will help your game, but serving yourself the right foods and vitamins will help *you*!

SUGGESTED SUPPLEMENT PROGRAM

- MVP, A.M. and P.M.
- Stress B complex with zinc, 1–3 times daily
- Chelated calcium, 750 mg., 1–3 times daily
- Vitamin E (dry form), 400–1,000 IU, daily
- Wheat germ oil

50. Racquetball Players

Since the 1970s, racquetball has become increasingly popular among fitness-conscious Americans. It's a game that can keep your whole body in motion, even when practicing by yourself. (If you are practicing, break up your hour into fifteen- to twenty-minute segments to prevent boredom and to keep yourself in motion.)

Professional racquetball players, such as Lynn Adams,

spend at least one and one half hours daily conditioning themselves (cycling, running, lifting weights) just to meet the demands of the game. For amateurs, warm-ups and cool-downs (see sections 23 and 26) are sufficient to increase flexibility and help prevent muscle injuries.

As with tennis, racquetball players should fortify themselves with a diet that is higher in complex carbohydrates than fats or protein. This will not only increase energy but will also allow you to lose body fat without losing necessary muscle tissue. (Without sufficient carbohydrates, the body can deplete muscle to get its needed fuel.)

SUGGESTED SUPPLEMENT PROGRAM

- MVP, A.M. and P.M.
- Stress B complex with zinc, 1–3 times daily
- Vitamin E (dry form), 400–1,000 IU, daily
- Chelated calcium, 750 mg., 1–3 times daily
- Cytochrome-C, inosine, and octacosanol, 1,000 mcg., 1–3 times daily

51. Body Builders

Lifting weights can help strengthen and tone your body, but even if you work continuously with weights—or even move from machine to machine quickly—you're not reaping great aerobic benefits.

What you have to keep in mind is that you *can't* convert fat to muscle. (Aerobic exercise is the only way to burn off fat. See section 10.) On the other hand, weight lifting can define and tone specific areas of the body. (This does *not* mean "spot reducing.") If you do work with weights, remember that muscles contract and need to be gently stretched, so warm-ups and cool-downs (see sections 23 and 26) are important.

Probably more important for body builders is being on the right diet. Without combining the two, you can wind up with bulging muscles, but they'll still be layered with fat, which won't do much for your overall shape.

Yes, it's true that proteins build and repair muscles, but it's complex carbohydrates that supply energy for the continuous and repeated muscular contractions that occur during prolonged exercise. For best results, I'd advise getting 80 to 90 percent of your calories from complex carbohydrates and no more than 10 percent from meat protein.

SUGGESTED SUPPLEMENT PROGRAM

- MVP, A.M. and P.M.
- Stress B complex with zinc, 1–3 times daily
- Vitamin E (dry form), 400–1,000 IU, 1–3 times daily
- Cytochrome-C, inosine, and octacosanol, 1,000 mcg., 1–3 times daily

52. Calisthenics and Gymnastics

Calisthenics (such as sit-ups, push-ups, jumping jacks, cartwheels, somersaults, and so on, where no apparatus is used) and gymnastics (such as feats performed on parallel bars, pommel horse, rings, balance beams, and so on) are the basis of physical education for most of the world.

The object of physical education is to introduce a balanced and graduated system of exercises to children in the early grades, going on to more advanced programs in high schools and colleges.

Unfortunately, most of us forget these basics (unless aiming for the Olympics or other professional competitions) and all too often try to pick them up without being either physically or nutritionally prepared. You can't, after years of lethargy, just somersault your way to fitness—at least, not immediately. No matter how great you were in gym during your high school days, it's not advisable to jump right into calisthenics or gymnastics without preparing your body for it. (See sections 23 and 26.)

SUGGESTED SUPPLEMENT PROGRAM

- MVP, with breakfast and dinner
- Vitamin B complex with zinc, 1–3 times daily
- Vitamin E (dry form), 200–400 IU, twice daily
- Cytochrome-C, inosine, and octacosanol, 1,000 mcg., 1–3 times daily

53. Yoga

Yoga is a series of remarkable exercises that not only can increase your flexibility and endurance and thus prepare you for numerous other activities, but also, if practiced on a regular basis, can benefit you in all areas of fitness—emotional, physical, and sexual.

> For warm-up, cool-down, and stress-relieving exercise, yoga can't be beat.

Yoga exercises are not meant to be strenuous (no whipping the body into shape here). They are designed to rest rather than exhaust the body; nonetheless, they offer phenomenal fitness rewards.

The premise of yoga is that most illness is caused by wrong posture, wrong mental attitudes, and wrong diet, which is why its basic precept is vegetarianism. Personally, I am not in favor of *total* vegetarianism, and don't feel that it is essential, on a fitness level, for engaging in these exercises. But if you are a vegetarian, I strongly advise the following supplements.

SUGGESTED SUPPLEMENT PROGRAM

- MVP, A.M. and P.M.
- Stress B complex with folic acid and zinc, 1–3 times daily
- Vitamin B_{12}, sublingual (cobalamin), 1–3 times daily
- Extra vitamin C is recommended. This should be taken with meals because it makes needed dietary iron more readily available, and fiber (a vegetarian staple) inhibits iron absorption.

54. Any Questions About Chapter II?

I'm a swimmer. I wash my hair every time I get out of the pool because I know chlorine can damage it, but the condition of my hair seems to be getting worse. Have you any nutritional suggestions that could help?

Quite a few. (See section 97 for a detailed regimen.) Meanwhile, check the ingredients on the shampoos you're using and make sure they contain no petrochemicals, such as propylparaben (which is much like chlorine and can dry out hair), methylparaben, propylene glycol or sodium lauryl sulfate. You want a shampoo without added synthetics. There are several on the market designed especially for swimmers. Check with your pharmacist or ask at your local health food supply store.

What's your feeling about the anabolic drugs that have recently been prescribed for athletes?

I'm not in favor of any drugs unless they're prescribed for specific medical reasons. HGH (human growth hormone) can definitely help athletic performance because of its anabolic (muscle-building) action, but the pituitary gland can be stimulated to produce its own HGH with natural supplements. (See section 63.)

The drugs being marketed now by European manufacturers under the trade names Crescormon and Asellacrin have FDA approval only for long-term treatment of dwarfism in children with a specific hormone deficiency. Besides, all the side effects of these drugs are still not known, though high blood pressure, acne, swollen nipples, and symptoms similar to diabetes have already been noted. I'd recommend avoiding these anabolics, at least until more is known about their contraindications.

As a runner, I perspire heavily. Does this mean I should increase the salt in my diet, or should I take salt supplements?

Neither! The average American eats at least sixty times the salt required by the body. Additionally, salt tablets have a dehydrating effect. They can cause cramping, gastrointestinal upsets, and can be a contributing factor to heat stroke. Your body knows how to conserve needed salt. In *rare* cases where there is a salt deficiency, the salt—a pinch— should be mixed in a solution of drinking water and sipped slowly.

I'm a semiprofessional tennis player, and, I believe, nutritionally fit. Nonetheless, I'd like to know if there are any supplements now available that I might not be aware of that could improve my game.

I'd say bee pollen. It's one of the most energizing supplements for competitive sports players, and an excellent source of vitamins (all of the B complex), minerals, protein, and natural gonadotropic and steroid hormone substances. It essentially balances your metabolism, increasing your endurance, and allows you to employ your skills to their maximum potential.

Last week at the gym I heard some of the guys talking about something called DMG. Is it a new drug? What does it do? And is it safe?

It's not new and it's not a drug. It can increase oxygen utilization for runners and reduce cramp-causing lactic acid buildup in muscles during exercise—and it's safe.

Actually, DMG (dimethylglycine) is the active constituent in pangamic acid and is essentially what was formerly known as vitamin B_{15}. Manufactured in our bodies from choline, it's used with other compounds in the production of hormones, enzymes, and nucleic acids essential for cell growth and repair. It works best when taken in conjunction with vitamins A and E.

Regaining Muscle Tone

If a person who regularly works out becomes sedentary, he will lose about 1 percent of muscle strength per day. Once exercise is resumed, however, retrieval of muscle tone takes *half that time*.

Marianne Battistone
Movement Therapist

Think about it . . .

III.

Dieting Fitness

55. Why Dieters Lose More Willpower Than Pounds

That most diets fail in the long run is a fact, but why they do continues to be a subject of controversy.

The "setpoint" theory is one of the most widely accepted today. It holds that fatness is caused by the setting of an area in the hypothalamus (part of the brain), sometimes referred to as an appestat, which controls your appetite for food. Obviously, everyone's appestat is not on the same setting.

> You can stay trimmer by moving more than by eating less!

According to recent research, the amount of fat cells you have, which were acquired at birth, craves more fat when the stores in these cells fall below a certain level. (The notion—popular a few years ago—that overfed infants would produce extra fat cells has now been rejected by most scientists, who feel that heredity is the major determinant.)

Glycerol, which is bound and released according to the fat content of a cell, along with the blood level of insulin, informs the brain of the body's fat reserves and sets your appestat accordingly. Great in theory, but, unfortunately, external influences can also affect your body's appestat. The aroma and taste of delectable food, for instance, can *raise* your appestat.

Certain drugs, such as amphetamines—and the nicotine in cigarettes—can lower your appestat. But once the pills or cigarettes are discontinued, your appestat goes right back up to where it was—and the weight returns.

Frustrating? You bet it is. But success is still attainable. The good news is that regular exercise and effective physical conditioning can *lower* your appestat! In other words, you can stay trimmer by moving more than by eating less. Instead of the temporary and potentially dangerous weight loss you get with pills or cigarettes, you can safely drop pounds, keep them off, and—with the right exercises and nutrients—become physically fit at the same time!

56. How You Can Reset Your Setpoint

Exercise! That's right, exercising regularly can reset the setpoint mechanism of the brain and help reduce your appetite by lowering the point at which you feel full.

To reset for weight loss, the minimum requirement is half an hour of aerobic exercise three times a week.

Physical activity stimulates metabolism for a number of hours after an exercise is completed. This is important for dieters to keep in mind because the body's natural response to a decreased food intake is to burn *fewer* calories. Exercise, therefore, not only can change your diet future, but your figure as well.

57. What You Should Weigh

Before rushing into the stress of a diet, I'd advise looking over the table below to see what the American Medical Association feels is the right weight for you. (I realize that the chart below will probably not satisfy the often outrageous cosmetic demands that models, actors, dancers, media personalities, and so forth put on their bodies, but if you're in the AMA's range, you should consider yourself healthy—and lucky.)

HEIGHT	HEALTHY WEIGHT (WITHOUT CLOTHES)		
	SMALL FRAME	AVERAGE FRAME	LARGE FRAME
MEN			
5'4"	122	133	145
5'6"	130	142	155
5'8"	139	151	166
5'10"	147	157	174
6'	154	169	183
6'2"	162	175	192
6'3"	165	178	195
WOMEN			
5'	100	109	118
5'2"	107	115	125
5'4"	113	122	132
5'6"	120	129	139
5'8"	126	136	146
5'10"	133	144	156
6'	141	152	166

58. How To Gain Fitness and Lose Fat

Calories burned up by exercise vary according to body weight. In half an hour's time, the heavier you are, the more calories you're going to use while indulging in any activity.

WEIGHT	ACTIVITY	CALORIES BURNED IN HALF AN HOUR
110–120 lbs.	Running	309–336
	Swimming	268–293
	Walking	206–225
	Fonda workout	227–248
	Cross-country skiing	351–383
	Cycling	289–315
	Skating	268–293
	Rowing	351–383
130–140 lbs.	Running	366–394
	Swimming	317–341
	Walking	244–263
	Fonda workout	269–289
	Cross-country skiing	414–446
	Cycling	341–368
	Skating	317–341
	Rowing	414–446
150–160 lbs.	Running	422–450
	Swimming	366–390
	Walking	281–300
	Fonda workout	309–330
	Cross-country skiing	478–510
	Skating	366–390
	Rowing	428–510

59. Foods to Increase

If fit and trim is what you want to be, then fiber foods are for you. What you have to be aware of, though, is that all fiber is not the same and that different types perform different functions.

Cellulose and Hemicellulose fiber foods	Whole wheat flour, bran, cabbage, young peas, green beans, wax beans, broccoli, brussels sprouts, cucumber skins, peppers, apples, carrots, whole grains, cereals, mustard greens, and beet roots

These absorb water and can smooth functioning of the large bowel. They "bulk" waste, moving it through the colon more rapidly, preventing constipation and also offering protection against diverticulosis, spastic colon, hemorrhoids, cancer of the colon, and varicose veins.

Gums and pectin	Oatmeal and other rolled oat products, dried beans, apples, citrus fruits, carrots, cauliflower, cabbage, dried peas, green beans, potatoes, squash, and strawberries

These primarily influence absorption in the stomach and small bowel. By binding with bile acids, they *decrease* fat absorption and lower cholesterol levels. By coating the lining of the gut, they delay stomach-emptying and thereby slow sugar absorption after a meal.

Lignin fiber	Bran, breakfast cereals, eggplant, green beans, strawberries, pears, radishes, and older vegetables (as vegetables age, their lignin content rises)

Lignin fiber foods reduce the digestibility of other fibers, lower cholesterol, and speed food through the gut.

CAUTION: High-fiber foods are great for energy and weight reduction, but too much in your diet can cause gas, bloating, nausea, vomiting, diarrhea, and possibly interfere with the body's ability to absorb such necessary minerals as zinc, calcium, iron, magnesium, and vitamin B_{12}. Fortunately, this can be easily prevented by varying your diet along with your high-fiber foods.

60. Foods to Decrease

If you're into shaping up, you definitely want to decrease your intake of refined carbohydrates, sugar, salt, and fat.

The following are some popular foods you should unpopularize in your diet:

Potato chips, cakes, cookies, carbonated soft drinks, chocolate, candy bars, chewing gum, sugared cereals; processed luncheon meats—hot dogs, Spam, bacon, bologna; Big Macs (each contains approximately 33 *grams of fat, 6 grams of sugar, and 963 mg. of sodium*); Burger King Whoppers (*41 grams of fat, 9 grams of sugar, and 1,083 mg. of sodium*); fast-food shakes (*8–14 teaspoons of sugar and 276–685 mg. of salt!*) and fries; ketchup (which has 8 percent more sugar than ice cream), soy sauce, butter, all animal fats

NOTE: Remember that protein does *not* mean nonfattening. The best reducing-high-energy diets should contain proportionately larger amounts of complex carbohydrates than protein and fat.

61. Salads Can Be Sneaky

Fruits and vegetables are great nutritional staples and snacks, but, like friends, you should select them carefully.

For example, it's true that an avocado offers a fine 580 IU of vitamin A, along with substantial amounts of potassium, calcium, and magnesium, among other nutrients—but it also contains 334 calories and a whopping 32.8 *grams* of fat! One large raw carrot, on the other hand, can give you a dazzling 11,000 IU of vitamin A, along with substantial amounts of other vitamins and minerals, but contains only 42 calories and .2 grams of fat.

All vegetables are not dieters' friends.

So if it's a toss-up between what you're going to put in the salad bowl, I'd advise checking out the food composition of your options. You can do this by writing to the U.S. Department of Agriculture, U.S. Government Printing Office, Washington, D.C. 20402 for *Composition of Foods*, Agriculture Handbook No. 8. It will tell you everything you need to know. (Prices of government books vary yearly, so you might want to query them first. *Composition of Foods* shouldn't be more than $5.00, and it's well worth the price.)

62. Diet Saboteurs

Have you ever wondered why you can't lose weight? Well, it could be because of what I call the diet saboteurs. These are those seemingly innocent substances in foods *and medicines* that the average person never thinks of as having anything to do with weight gain.

SUGAR

Let's take that cream substitute you use in your coffee. It's 65 percent sugar! A chocolate bar is only 51 percent sugar! Hidden sugars are where you least expect them, which is why I always stress reading labels. Be on the lookout for words ending in "-ose," which indicates the presence of sugar. By any other name, a sugar is still a sugar. In fact, even medicines can be fattening.

MEDICINES	SUGAR PER TABLESPOON
Alternagel Liquid	2,000 mg.
Basaljel Extra-strength Liquid	375 mg.
Gaviscon Liquid	1,500 mg.
Gaviscon-2 tablets	2,400 mg.
Maalox plus tablets	575 mg.
Mylanta Liquid	2,000 mg.
Riopan Plus Chew tablets	610 mg.

SALT

This is not only a diet saboteur, but an isidious health depleter. The normal intake of sodium chloride (table salt) is 6 to 18 g. daily; an intake over 14 g. is considered excessive. Well, far too many of us are excessive without even knowing it. (The average American consumes about fifteen pounds—a bowling ball—of salt each year!)

Too much salt can cause high blood pressure, increase your chances of heart disease, cause abnormal fluid retention and migraine headaches, deplete potassium, and interfere with proper utilization of protein foods.

Keeping away from pretzels, snack foods, and that shaker on the table helps, but salt traps are as hidden from view as sugar ones.

KNOW THOSE SALT TRAPS:

- Beer (there's 25 mg. of sodium in every 12 ounces).
- Baking soda, MSG (monosodium glutamate), and baking powder.
- Laxatives (check labels, most contain high amounts of sodium).
- Home water softeners (they add sodium to the water, so whether you're drinking it or cooking with it, you're getting more than you want).
- When reading labels, aside from the words "salt" and "sodium," be on the lookout for the chemical symbol *Na*.
- Cured meats—ham, bacon, corned beef, frankfurters, sausage—shellfish or any canned or frozen meat, poultry, or fish to which sodium has been added.
- Diet sodas! The calories might be low, but the sodium content is *high*!
- Club sodas. (An 8 oz. glass of Canada Dry club soda has 75 mg. of sodium!) My advice: Get your soda fizz from salt-free seltzer.

MEDICATIONS THAT CAUSE WEIGHT GAIN OR BLOATING

- Anticoagulants (blood thinners)
- Antidepressants
- Anti-inflammatories/antiarthritics
- Antispasmodics/anticholinergics (stomach and cramp pills)
- Oral contraceptives, estrogens, and progestogens (birth control pills and sex hormones)

- Tranquilizers, sedatives, relaxants, barbiturates, and hypnotics
- Antidyskinetics (used for treatment of Parkinson's disease)

63. How To Eat a Little More and Gain a Lot Less

Supplement your diet with arginine and ornithine.

Remember when you were a kid and could eat all you wanted without gaining weight? Well, that was because your pituitary gland was still producing HGH, human growth hormone. Unfortunately, as we grow older, growth hormone production falls off and the pounds pile on.

> You can rejuvenate your metabolism while you sleep.

The amino acids arginine and ornithine, available as supplements, have been found to stimulate the pituitary gland to continue to produce growth hormone. In effect, by using these supplements, you can rejuvenate your metabolism, and they'll work while you sleep because that's when growth hormone is secreted.

It's true that some hormones encourage the body to store fat, but growth hormone acts as a mobilizer of fat, helping you not only to look trimmer but to have more energy as well. This doesn't mean you can pig out and stay slim, but you can certainly potentiate any diet and exercise regimen you're on.

SUPPLEMENT ADVICE

Arginine and ornithine supplements are available in tablets or powder and work best when taken on an empty stomach with water (no protein). For rejuvenating metabolism, take 2 grams (2,000 mg.) immediately before retiring. For muscle-toning benefits, take same dosage one hour prior to engaging in vigorous physical exercise.

CAUTION: Arginine is contraindicated for growing children, persons with schizophrenic conditions, and anyone who has a herpes virus infection. Doses exceeding 20–30 grams daily are *not* recommended. (These could cause enlarged joints and bone deformities.)

64. Other Natural Reducers

PHENYLALANINE

This essential amino acid is a neurotransmitter, a chemical that transmits signals between nerve cells and the brain. In the body it's turned into norepinephrine and dopamine, excitatory transmitters, which promote alertness and vitality, *and* reduce hunger.

For appetite control, phenylalanine, available in 250–500 mg. tablets, should be taken one hour before meals with water (no protein).

CAUTION: Though a natural substance, phenylalanine is contraindicated during pregnancy and for anyone with skin cancer or PKU (phenylketonuria). It can raise blood pressure, so hypertensives or anyone with a heart condition should check with a doctor before using phenylalanine.

CCK (CHOLECYSTOKININ)

This polypeptide hormone, which also functions as a brain neurotransmitter, seems to act as a satiety ("I am full!") signal in the body. (A possible resetter of the setpoint.) It is now on the market in supplement form. Two 1,000 mg. tablets should be taken one half hour before meals with a full glass of water, for best effects.

L-phenylalanine is a potent releaser of CCK. (L-phenylalanine is the natural form; D-phenylalanine is the synthetic form and does *not* release CCK.)

Vitamin B$_6$ and vitamin C, taken with L-phenyl-alanine, potentiate the release of CCK.

SPIRULINA

Aside from containing very high-quality protein and virtually all the vitamins and minerals you need, this blue-green algae, known as spirulina plankton, contains phenylalanine, which, as noted above, acts on the brain's appetite center to decrease hunger. Spirulina also keeps blood sugar at the proper level, eliminating those dangerous cravings for unnecessary snacks.

CAUTION: Not approved for treatment of diabetes unless medically prescribed.

Available in 500 mg. tablets as well as in powder form, spirulina works best when taken one half hour before meals. Start with three 500 mg. tablets before each meal and then decrease to two or one. (In rare cases, an individual might require six to eight tablets before meals to obtain initial benefits.)

GLUCOMANNAN

Found in konjak root, glucomannan is one of the best dietary plant fibers available. Because it is *not* digested by the body, it helps you reduce as it passes through the digestive tract. It helps control appetite, promotes improved metabolism, and accelerates the burning of excess fat.

Also, because it can impede the digestion of fats, it alleviates hunger pangs during dieting and can help prevent constipation.

Glucomannan should be taken half an hour to one hour before a meal (average adult dosage is 500–1,500 mg.) with one to two glasses of water. If your stomach is easily upset, take glucomannan after eating.

CAUTION: If you are on a fiber-restricted diet, do *not* use this product without checking with your doctor. If rash or other allergic symptoms develop, discontinue use.

GTF (GLUCOSE TOLERANCE FACTOR)

Derived from chromium-rich brewer's yeast, GTF supplements help regulate blood sugar levels and are therefore useful for dieters in suppressing hunger.

An average supplemental dose for adults would be 200–600 mcg. daily.

CAUTION: Not approved for treatment of diabetes unless medically prescribed.

65. Dangerous Diets

The Cambridge and liquid protein diets are not only dangerous, they're potentially lethal. (The liquid protein diet is no longer on the market.) Radical diets such as these (where the daily caloric intake is between 330 and

600) can cause abnormal heart function and severe deficiencies in vital minerals due to extremely rapid weight loss. They should *never* be undertaken without strict medical supervision.

Any diet that excludes an entire group of nutrients, such as carbohydrates as advised by Dr. Robert C. Atkins for the first week of his carbohydrate-restricted regimen, is not recommended for fitness. Without carbohydrates, your body can't burn fat efficiently, and also toxic by-products called "ketones" are produced. The result is supposed to force the body to draw upon stored fats for fuel, but more often than not, muscles are depleted of energy.

If you intend to shape up, don't shortchange your body. (See section 70, Mindell's Fired-for-Fitness Diet.)

66. Don't Put Off for Tomorrow What You Should Be Putting on Today

ADVICE FOR THE UNDERWEIGHT

With so many people driving themselves daily to lose weight, it's difficult to imagine that there are many others trying just as desperately to gain weight. In fact, putting *on* weight can often be more difficult than taking it off.

If you're slightly underweight, but still look and feel great and have lots of vitality, you have nothing to worry about. But if you tire easily, are nervous or high strung, and often succumb to illness, you're what is often referred to medically as the "asthenic" type—extremely frail and not physically fit.

If you're planning a weight-gaining program, don't go for quick empty-calorie foods such as candies, ice cream, cakes, and so forth. What your body needs are nutritious calorie-rich pound increasers, foods that will not only increase your weight but your energy as well.

> Don't start by scaring your stomach with too much food.

Gorging yourself with banana splits, milk shakes, or excessive amounts of any food is a bad way to begin. If you want success, you don't want to scare your stomach with an onslaught it's unprepared for. Easy-eating, high-calorie, high-nutrition meals and snacks are the way to go.

SOME GREAT PUT ONS

Avocados

Just one gives you 334 calories and lots of nutrients. (Mash one into guacamole and enjoy it with ½ cup —246 calories—of sour cream.)

Sweet potatoes

You get 155 calories for the potato and an extra 100 if you top it with a tablespoon of butter, to say nothing of the 9,230 IU of vitamin A, and substantial amounts of vitamin C, potassium, and calcium.

Dates

Snack on 10 a day and you'll add 274 calories to your intake, while benefiting from 648 mg. of potassium, while helping to fill your daily requirement for calcium and magnesium.

Raisins

Sprinkle them on salads and snack on them for fun because ½ cup adds 230

	calories to your diet and supplies you with fine amounts of calcium and magnesium.
Cheese	Go for it! Top desserts with it, use it for snacks, make your own pizza and double up the cheese on it! Make lasagna with lots of whole milk ricotta—1 cup has 428 calories and more than half your daily requirement of calcium.
Go nuts	Roasted almonds have 984 calories a cup, peanuts have 836. Just 6 macadamia nuts will add on 109 calories! And don't forget about pumpkin and sesame seeds, which can flesh you out per cup at 774 and 873 calories respectively. And best of all, they're good for you!

TIPS

- For liquids, go for juice instead of water. (Prune juice has 200 calories per 8 ounces.)
- Garnish vegetables with a dollop of sour cream or mayonnaise.
- Use honey or blackstrap molasses for sweeteners on breakfast cereals. (And don't skip breakfast!)
- Relax with a late-night snack. A white-meat turkey sandwich, with mayo, and a glass of milk will give you calories and the natural tranquilizer tryptophan.
- To improve your appetite, I'd recommend the following supplements:
    - Vitamin B complex, 50–100 mg., taken with each meal

- Vitamin B$_{12}$, 2,000 mcg. (sublingual), with breakfast
- An organic iron complex tablet (containing vitamin C, copper, liver, manganese, and zinc to help assimilate iron)

• Select an exercise that won't overtire you, but will help you relieve tension. (See section 53 on yoga.) Just because you're putting on weight doesn't mean it has to go to all the wrong places.

67. There's Nothing Lightweight About Anorexia

Victims become physically unable to eat and literally starve themselves to death.

Anorexia nervosa is an eating disorder characterized by a pathological lack of appetite that becomes so extreme that the victims of this illness become physically *unable* to eat and literally starve themselves to death.

Teenage girls seem to be most susceptible to anorexia nervosa, though it can happen at any age and to members of either sex. Psychologists believe that the self-starvation that is the hallmark of anorexia is a sort of desperate attempt on the part of the victim to gain independence and control of his or her life.

Anorexia and bulimia (which is characterized by a compulsive eating of enormous quantities of food, then purging it from the body through vomiting or laxatives) have become dangerously prevalent in our weight-conscious society. Psychotherapy has been shown to help many victims of these illnesses, but, unfortunately, many people afflicted with these ailments are not aware that they're in need of treatment.

YOU MIGHT NEED TREATMENT IF...

- your obsession with not gaining weight takes precedence over all other activities;
- your eating habits are irrational (in public you'll order a salad and then go home and wolf down every leftover in the refrigerator);
- you use laxatives as a vehicle for weight loss;
- you purge yourself by vomiting after meals;
- you eat junk foods in secret;
- you exercise compulsively after eating;
- no matter what weight charts say, you always feel too fat;
- you lie to others about what you have or have not eaten.

68. Who's Where: Feedback for Anorectics

If you feel—even vaguely—that you might have an eating disorder, you can write for help. Send a stamped, self-addressed envelope to any one the following organizations:

National Association of Anorexia Nervosa and
Associated Disorders
P.O. Box 271
Highland Park, IL 60035

National Anorexic Aid Society
P.O. Box 29461
Columbus, OH 43229 (They request a $1.00 donation.)

Associates for Bulimia and Related Disorders
31 West 10 Street
New York, NY 10011

69. Why Dieters Crave the Wrong Foods

Most diets restrict the intake of carbohydrates, regrettably not distinguishing between the good (complex carbohydrates) and the bad (refined sugars, candies, and so on). But because a low carbohydrate intake can decrease the level of serotonin in the brain (a chemical that can act as an appetite regulator), dieters feel hungry and crave the nutrient that can most rapidly elevate serotonin levels—carbohydrates.

> Cookies, ice cream, and candy become a dieter's downfall because they raise blood sugar levels.

Unfortunately, the most accessible and desirable carbohydrates are those that have been strictly prohibited. (Chocolate is often craved by dieters after a broken love affair because it contains phenylethylamine, a substance that the brain produces when you're in love, and craves when you fall out of it.)

Weight specialists now believe that there are specific carbohydrate receptors in the brain—and the heavier you are, the more you have. This means an increase in carbohydrate craving even after the appetite has been appeased with other foods.

Why cookies, ice cream, candy, and so forth become a dieter's downfall is because they can most rapidly raise blood sugar levels, which produces a tranquilizing effect. After a heavy sugar intake, insulin floods the system, and—despite the fact that it makes one sluggish—insulin increases the amount of the amino acid tryptophan entering the brain, which is necessary for the production of serotonin, the body's own tranquilizer.

My advice? Take a tryptophan supplement (250–500 mg. three times daily) between meals, with water, and avoid the high-caloric, sugar-insulin diet blues. It will keep your spirits up and your weight down.

70. Mindell's Fired-for-Fitness Diet

The following diet has been designed as a seven-day program that can provide you with enhanced energy and optimal weight loss at the same time.

CAUTION: Before starting this, or any diet, consult your doctor or a nutritionally oriented physician (see section 145). These regimens are recommendations, not prescriptions, and are not intended as medical advice, nor should they be construed to replace any specific instructions or warnings given to you by your doctor or a particular product's information sheet.

MONDAY   *Approx. Calorie Count: 1,205*

Breakfast

1 slice whole wheat bread
⅓ cup cottage cheese
½ cup skim (nonfat) milk
½ grapefruit

Lunch

1 slice whole wheat bread
3 oz. chicken
1 tsp. mayo
½ cup carrot strips, cuke, pepper

Dinner

3 oz. potato
3 oz. liver
½ cup broccoli
small green salad
2 tsp. oil with vinegar and garlic
small orange
½ cup skim milk

Snack
20 small grapes
1 cup skim milk

TUESDAY   *Approx. Calorie Count: 934*

Breakfast
1 oz. cereal (oatmeal, 100% bran, puffed wheat
   no sugar added)
1 cup skim milk
¼ melon—cantaloupe (or frozen melon balls, 1
   cup)

Lunch
2 slices rye bread
3 oz. water-pack tuna
1 tsp. mayo
small salad (lettuce, celery, cuke)
½ cup skim milk

Dinner
½ cup string beans
small green salad
2 tsp. oil with garlic and vinegar
3 oz. turkey
small tangerine

Snack
½ cup blueberries or strawberries
   mixed with ½ cup nonfat yogurt

WEDNESDAY   *Approx. Calorie Count: 1,120*

Breakfast
1 slice whole wheat bread
⅓ cup cottage cheese
½ cup skim milk
½ grapefruit

Lunch
2 eggs scrambled with 1 tsp. margarine
2 tbsp. onion
1 slice rye toast
½ cup unsweetened applesauce mixed with
   ½ cup yogurt

Dinner
Pasta Salad
   1 oz. uncooked or ⅔ cup cooked whole wheat
      pasta
   3 oz. chicken, shredded
   1 cup combination broccoli, cauliflower florets,
      mushrooms, scallions, tomato
         mix with 2 tsp. oil with garlic and vinegar
         serve hot or cold

Snack
¼ cantaloupe or 1 cup frozen melon balls
½ cup nonfat yogurt

THURSDAY

Approx. Calorie Count:
857 w/snapper
957 w/veal

Breakfast
small orange
1 oz. cereal
½ cup skim milk

Lunch
3 oz. tuna
small salad (lettuce, tomato, celery)
1 tsp. mayo
2 rye wafers (3½" long, 1⅞" wide, ¼" thick)
½ cup nonfat yogurt

Dinner
3 oz. red snapper (or
  3 oz. veal)
½ cup zucchini
small salad
2 tsp. oil with garlic and vinegar

Snack
small apple
1 cup skim milk

FRIDAY

Approx. Calorie Count: 1,074

Breakfast
¼ cantaloupe or 1 cup frozen melon balls
1 egg poached or boiled
1 slice whole wheat bread
1 tsp. margarine
1 cup skim milk

Lunch
⅔ cup cottage cheese (low-fat)
½ cup unsweetened fruit cocktail
1 slice whole wheat bread
1 tsp. margarine
1 small carrot
½ cup skim milk

Dinner
3 oz. sole (or similar fish)
1 tsp. margarine
½ cup broccoli
small tomato, sliced
3 oz. potato, baked

Snack
¼ med. pineapple or
   1 cup canned pineapple in own juice
½ cup nonfat yogurt
1 cup popcorn

SATURDAY   *Approx. Calorie Count: 1,203*

Breakfast
1 cup tomato juice
1 oz. cereal
½ cup milk

Lunch
3 oz. turkey   )
1 tsp. mayo   )
2 slices whole wheat bread)—turkey sandwich
lettuce   )
tomato, sliced   )

small carrot
½ cup applesauce unsweetened, mixed with
½ cup nonfat yogurt

Dinner
3 oz. chicken
½ cup green peas
½ cup brown rice
2 tsp. margarine

Snack
small orange
½ cup skim milk

SUNDAY   *Approx. Calorie Count: 1,100*

Breakfast
small orange
1 egg poached or boiled
1 slice whole-grain bread
½ cup nonfat yogurt

Lunch
2 oz. sliced mozzarella cheese (low-fat))
½ whole wheat muffin   )
small tomato, sliced   )—pizza
1 tsp. olive oil with oregano sprinkled   )
  on top
¼ cantaloupe or 1 cup frozen melon balls

Dinner
3 oz. halibut (or similar fish)
½ cup cauliflower
½ cup string beans
1 cup skim milk

Snack
½ banana mixed with
½ cup nonfat yogurt

71. Any Questions About Chapter III?

My sister-in-law has been on a diet for two months, lost fifteen pounds, and swears that she has eaten pasta every day. Could this be possible?

Absolutely. There are only 200 calories in a cup of pasta (providing it's not drenched in butter) and these burn slowly, giving a dieter lasting energy— along with protein, calcium, phosphorus, iron, and quite a few important B vitamins. The right carbohydrates at the right time can be a dieter's best friends.

You seem to be opposed to low-carbohydrate diets. Could you tell me why? Every time I've gone on one, I've lost weight.

But have you kept that weight off? Obviously not. The reason most people feel that low-carbohydrate diets work is because they alter your mineral metabolism and bring about a quick loss of body water. Sure, it looks great on the scale, but this sort of dehydration is short-lived and takes its toll on energy levels. I'm not opposed to low-carbohydrate diets *if* the carbohydrates being cut out are those that shouldn't be included in the first place— refined sugars, junk foods, and so on. It's those guys that have given carbohydrates a bad name.

What's so bad about taking diet drugs to help you reduce?

Aside from such possible side effects as insomnia, constipation (or diarrhea), dizziness, elevated blood pressure, heart palpitations, cerebral hemorrhage, seizures, and addiction, it's been shown that people taking these drugs regain weight much more quickly than those who diet without them. Though you might lose more weight initially with an appetite suppressant, the odds of trimming down in the long run are against you. Changing your eating habits and selecting the right foods (see section 59) are what you need to really shape up.

What is DIT?

Dietary-induced thermogenesis (DIT) is essentially a metabolic process that occurs after meals and increases the body's rate of burning calories. (Exercising a few hours after eating—not right after— will help you lose weight because calories are burned faster than on an empty stomach.)

It's not certain what triggers DIT, but it is known that carbohydrates are important to the process and lead to less storage of fat than the same amount of protein calories consumed. So, if you want to slim down, think twice about passing over the bun for the burger. Recent studies indicate that favoring meat over whole grains could substantially contribute to obesity.

I chew a lot of sugarless gum to keep my weight down. I know the gum doesn't contain saccharin, but it does have other artificial sweeteners. How safe are these?

Most sugarless gums and dietetic candies use mannitol and sorbitol as sweeteners. (These are absorbed slowly by the body, much like carbohydrates, and therefore have little effect on blood sugar levels.) As far as safety goes, neither of these sweeteners has been implicated as a carcinogen. On the other hand, both mannitol and sorbitol have been found to produce gas, bloating, cramps, and diarrhea.

TIME OUT

Why Thin People Get Fat

If you eat an additional 100 calories a day,
approximately the equivalent of
one of the following:

> 1 banana
> 1 large apple
> 1 tbsp. peanut butter
> 1 tbsp. mayonnaise
> 1 tbsp. butter or margarine
> 1 pack of Life Savers
> 1 jigger of 80 proof gin, rum, vodka,
>   or whiskey
> 1 large macaroon
> 1 scoop sherbet
> 1 glass of cola

you will gain 10 pounds a year.
In ten years, that's one hundred pounds!

Think about it . . .

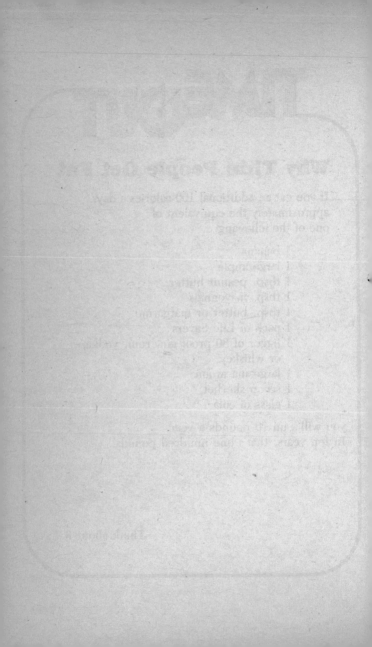

IV.

Pregnancy Shape-up

72. Get a Healthy Head Start

The time to think about shaping up for pregnancy is *before* you become pregnant! So, if you're contemplating parenthood, now is when you should go all-out for fitness.

DIET

If you are overweight, lose those pounds before conception. Obesity can cause numerous and often dangerous problems in the course of pregnancy—especially during labor and delivery—and trying to lose weight while you are pregnant is generally not advisable. Your chances for a healthier baby and a happier pregnancy are substantially greater if you are at your proper weight level when you conceive. (See section 57.)

Your pre-conception diet should include a plentiful variety of nutritious foods, particularly those rich in iron.

BEST IRON-RICH BETS	REWARDS
Liver (3 oz.)	7–12 mg.
Prune juice (1 cup)	10.5 mg.

Best Iron-Rich Bets	Rewards
Oysters (4 oz., raw)	6.2 mg.
Dried apricots (½ cup)	4.1 mg.
Asparagus spears (8 average, canned, drained)	3.0 mg.
Peas (1 cup, cooked)	2.9 mg.
Beet greens (1 cup, cooked)	2.8 mg.
Wheat germ (¼ cup)	2.5 mg.
Tofu (1 cake)	2.2 mg.

Vitamins C and E aid in the assimilation of iron, so be sure you're eating enough foods with these vitamins (see section 36) or taking supplements.

Keep your diet varied. Too much phosphorus can interfere with iron absorption unless your body is being supplied with sufficient calcium. (I'd advise taking a high-potency multiple vitamin and chelated multiple-mineral supplement with breakfast and dinner, just to keep your nutritional bases covered.) Also, keep away from coffee and tea. They, too, can interfere with iron absorption.

EXERCISE

The more physically fit you are before becoming pregnant, the better you'll be able to deal with the stresses of pregnancy. (Think of it as an athletic event, and prepare for it the same way.) Certain exercises are not recommended during pregnancy, but if your body has become used to working out, you'll be able to get a lot more from the exercises that have been designed for pregnant women.

DRUGS AND MEDICATIONS

- If you've been taking oral contraceptives, it's advisable to wait at least three months after discontinuing use to become pregnant.
- If you are on *any* medication at all, ask your doctor about the risks involved *before* attempting to conceive.
- Have a complete gynecological examination. (This is particularly important if you or your partner has—or has had—a venereal disease.) Be sure to tell the doctor that you're thinking of becoming pregnant as you might need immunization against rubella (German measles), in which case you'll probably be advised to postpone attempting conception for at least three months to avoid endangering your baby.

73. Overcoming Infertility

On the rise in America for the past forty years, infertility can be caused by any number of reasons and occurs in both sexes in roughly equal proportions.

Becoming aware of fertility potentiators and pitfalls has helped innumerable couples achieve conception without having to resort to extreme or expensive medical procedures.

FERTILITY PITFALLS

- Drugs that lower sperm counts, such as:
  Azulfidine (sulfasalazine)—an anti-infective medication usually used in the control of diseases such as enteritis or colitis
  Bactrim, Septra (sulfamethoxazole and trimethoprim) —sulfonamides commonly prescribed for urinary tract infections

Colsalide Improved (colchicine)—an antiuric acid, antigout drug

Tagamet (cimetidine)—a drug used frequently in the treatment of ulcers

Phenobarbital—a barbiturate that's used as a hypnotic, sedative, and anticonvulsant

Marijuana—though this illicit drug is often thought safe by users, it has been found to lower sperm counts in heavy smokers.

- Oral contraceptives. If these are taken over a long period of time, they can cause irregular—even suppressed—ovulation after they've been discontinued.
- Intrauterine devices (IUDs). Women who use IUDs for contraception have a greater risk of pelvic inflammatory disease, which can result in damage to the fallopian tubes.
- Lack of sufficient nutrients in the diet, particularly vitamins B_2 (riboflavin), E, iron, and zinc.

FERTILITY POTENTIATORS

- Vitamin C, 500–1,000 mg., twice daily, has been found to substantially reduce clumping, or agglutination of sperm in the semen, a common cause of infertility.
- Natural fruits, such as bananas, which contain fructose, can nourish sperm production.
- Vitamin E (dry form), 200–400 mg., 1–3 times daily can be a fertility potentiator for males and females.
- Ginseng, taken either in capsule or liquid form, or drunk as a tea, over a period of time, appears to improve fertility.
- Zinc, chelated, 50 mg., 1–2 times daily can also help. (Remember that zinc works best with vitamin A, calcium, and phosphorus, so see section 36 to be sure that foods containing those nutrients are in your diet.)

Taking a supplement of vitamin B$_6$ with your zinc is advised to maximize its fertility potential.

74. Home Pregnancy Tests Don't Have All the Answers

Home pregnancy tests, which are available over the counter at most pharmacies, are based on the detection of human chorionic gonadotrophin (HCG) in a woman's urine. HCG is a hormone that's produced by the early developing placenta, released into the bloodstream, and then excreted into the urine.

Though it's possible to detect pregnancy as early as six days after conception, home pregnancy kits recommend waiting six to nine days after a missed menstrual period for testing. Instructions, chemicals, and equipment are provided; all you need do is supply a specimen of your first morning urine. The FDA apparently has no qualms about the manufacturers' claims of 95 to 98 percent accuracy for these tests, but *you* should be aware of factors that can contribute to inaccuracy.

Inaccurate results can occur . . .
- if the test is performed—or results evaluated—too early;
- if urine and/or chemicals are exposed to extreme temperatures;
- if you have a urinary tract infection or recently completed taking medication for one;
- if test equipment has been washed with soap (which could leave a residue and alter results);
- if there are excessive amounts of protein in your urine;
- if your pregnancy is ectopic (implantation occurs outside the uterus, most often the fallopian tube).

CAUTION: Ectopic pregnancies can be dangerous. If you suspect that you're pregnant and get negative results on your home test, I strongly recommend you see your doctor as soon as possible.

• if you are on any medication, especially birth control pills, antihypertensives, or tranquilizers, which can produce false positive results;
• if you have uterine cancer.

CAUTION: Getting a positive result on your test should encourage you to see a doctor as soon as possible, not put the visit off.

In all cases, a follow-up examination by a qualified physician is strongly recommended to protect your health—and your baby's.

75. Teenage Pregnancies Require Special Shape-ups

Teenage mothers have greater nutritional needs than women who have already completed their adult growth. Dietary iron is usually low in young women, and the stress of pregnancy can lead to anemia. Also, teenage mothers often have low calcium levels, which, if uncorrected, can endanger both mother and baby.

Because of nutritional inadequacies, teenage mothers are prone to toxemia or eclampsia (toxemia of pregnancy), which is a retention of fluids that can be extremely dangerous to both mother and baby, and is usually characterized by a marked elevation in blood pressure. This is a serious pregnancy risk, and requires immediate attention. (Early treatment, though, which is most often bed rest and sodium restriction, can usually alleviate the problem.) Also, the newborns of teenage mothers are generally below normal weight.

In addition to the regular increased nutritional needs

during pregnancy (see section 76), a teenage mother-to-be should add two cups of milk (or nutritional equivalent) to her diet and try to maintain a protein intake of 100 grams daily.

The following foods should be included in a teenage mother's diet: liver, meat, egg yolks, asparagus, oatmeal, milk, cheese, green vegetables, whole grains, dried beans, salmon, and sardines.

76. Just Because Your Nutritional Needs Increase Doesn't Mean You Have To Become a Blimp

It's true that during pregnancy the body's demand for vitamins increases. Just keep in mind that vitamins don't mean calories!

No matter how happy a woman is about being pregnant, there is always stress involved: worries about whether the child will be healthy, whether there will be enough money to pay the bills, whether you'll have to leave your job, and so on. And these stresses take their toll on mother and fetus.

The body responds to stress by producing more adrenal hormones. These provide the extra energy that's necessary when action is called for. But if there's no physical outlet for the energy, it's redirected to the digestive or nervous system or to some other organ system. In many instances, this is what's responsible for pregnancy fatigue, headaches, insomnia, and morning sickness. But, more important, this accelerated adrenal hormone production revs up the metabolism to such a degree that stores of valuable calcium are depleted, along with protein, phosphorus, and potassium, which are rapidly excreted just when the growing fetus needs them most.

PREGNANT WOMEN NEED A MINIMUM OF:

DAILY REQUIREMENT

During Pregnancy		For Nursing Mothers
74–76 g. protein daily		add 10
6,000 IU	Vitamin A	add 200
400–500 IU	Vitamin D	same
80–100 IU	Vitamin E	add 10
80–100 mg.	Vitamin C	add 20
1.5 mg.	Vitamin B_1	add 0.1 mg.
1.5 mg.	Vitamin B_2	add 0.2 mg.
2.6 mg.	Vitamin B_6	add 0.1 mg.
8–10 mcg.	Vitamin B_{12}	same
800 mcg.	Folic Acid	subtract 300 mcg.
16 mg.	Niacin	add 3 mg.
1,200 mg.	Calcium*	same
1,200 mg.	Phosphorus	same
450 mg.	Magnesium	same
30–60 mg.	Supplemental iron	same
175 mcg.	Iodine	add 25 mcg.
20 mg.	Zinc	add 5 mg.

*Don't use calcium tablets as a replacement for milk unless directed to do so by a doctor.

But despite your increased nutritional needs, you don't have to select the foods with the highest caloric content to fill them.

Setting the standard: 1 cup of whole milk equals 159 calories, 8.5 g. protein, 225 mg. phosphorus, 351 mg. potassium, and 291 mg. calcium.

Let's Talk Low-Calorie, High-Nutrition Alternatives

Food	Calories	Protein	Phosphorus	Potassium	Calcium
½ cup instant nonfat dried milk	122	11.8 g.	335 mg.	580 mg.	418 mg.
½ cup ricotta cheese	170	14.0 g.	228 mg.	154 mg.	334 mg.
½ cup cottage cheese (2% fat)	101	15.0 g.	170 mg.	108 mg.	77 mg.
salmon, ½ cup pink, canned	155	22.5 g.	314 mg.	387 mg.	265 mg.
shrimp, ½ lb. fresh	206	41.0 g.	376 mg.	499 mg.	143 mg.
cantaloupe, ¼ average	30	.7 g.	16 mg.	251 mg.	14 mg.
½ cup collard greens, cooked	21	1.9 g.	28 mg.	169 mg.	110 mg.
2 slices whole wheat bread	110	4.8 g.	104 mg.	136 mg.	46 mg.

By mixing and matching these foods in various combinations and dishes, you can maximize your nutritional intake and minimize weight gain.

NOTE: Shrimp is high in cholesterol—340 mg. per ½ lb.—so it's not advised for those who must keep their cholesterol levels down. But shellfish do have redeeming features, namely, 95 mg. magnesium and 453 mg. zinc!

77. A Pregnant Woman's Guide to Medicines

No drug—whether it's OTC or prescription, alcohol, nicotine, or caffeine—should be considered safe during pregnancy! Most drugs can cross the placenta and affect your unborn baby as well as you.

Considering that the major stages in an embryo's development occur during the first few weeks of life, before most women even *know* that they're pregnant, it's wise, if you're even *contemplating* motherhood, to think twice and check with a physician before taking *any medicine*!

Aspirin or salicylate analgesics, such as Anacin, Bufferin, Alka Seltzer, and so on, especially if overused in the third trimester, may prolong pregnancy or labor and cause severe bleeding in both mother and newborn before, during, and after delivery.

Antacids, such as Maalox, Milk of Magnesia, Camalox, Rolaids, and others, should not be taken for prolonged periods, or in high doses. They may cause muscle problems in the fetus, and sodium antacids can cause a pregnant woman to retain too much water.

Anticough medicines, such as terpin hydrate products, contain large amounts of alcohol, which can cause birth defects. (Be aware of how much more alcohol you're adding to your daily intake.)

Diuretics, such as Hygroton, Hydro-Diuril, Lasix, and

others, if used routinely, can be dangerous to mother and fetus, and may cause liver and/or blood disorders in newborns.

Antidiarrheals containing paragoric, if used too often, may lead to drug dependency in newborns and cause withdrawal symptoms. (If taken just prior to delivery, these medications have been known to cause breathing problems in newborns.)

Prescription antinausea preparations containing doxylamine with pyridoxine might cause birth defects.

Topical hydrocortisone products, such as Anusol-HC, used for the treatment of hemorrhoids can, if used in large amounts or for prolonged periods, be absorbed through the skin and cause birth defects.

Tetracyclines, especially if used in the last half of pregnancy, may cause discoloration of forming teeth in newborns as well as retard their teeth and bone growth.

Decongestants containing pseudoephedrine may cause a reduction in size and rate of bone formation in the fetus.

Laxatives, such as bulk-forming Serutan or Effersyllium, which contain large amounts of sodium or sugar may increase blood pressure and cause water retention. Saline laxatives—Epsom Salts, Citrate of Magnesia, Phospho-Soda—containing magnesium or potassium should be avoided if your kidney functions are not normal; those containing sodium should be avoided if you tend to retain water. Repeated use of mineral oil as a laxative can decrease proper absorption of foods, vitamins, and oral medications. It may also cause blood disorders in newborns. Castor oil can also be dangerous because it may cause contractions in the womb.

Quinine, which is available OTC, may cause birth defects and stimulate premature labor.

Tranquilizers and sedatives, such as Seconal, Phenobarbital, Librium, Valium, Dalmane, and others,
may increase chances of birth defects. These drugs
can also cause dependency and withdrawal symptoms in newborns. (Used late in pregnancy or during labor, they have been known to cause breathing
problems in newborns.) Phenothiazine products—
Thorazine, Compazine, Phenergan—are also not
recommended as they can cause jaundice and muscle tremors in newborns.

78. Natural Remedies for Pregnancy Discomforts

Along with the joys of prospective motherhood there are
often attendant discomforts. Before rushing off for a
prescription or an over-the-counter preparation with ingredients that might be more harmful than helpful, why
not go for relief in ways that have proven themselves
effective naturally?

IMPORTANT: *Your individual condition might preclude
the use of certain foods or vitamins that are suggested.
Please be aware that these regimens, along with others in
the book, are not prescriptive nor intended as medical
advice, and should be discussed with your doctor.*

NAUSEA

The changes in your body hormone levels, low
blood sugar, digestive slowdown, and often not enough B
vitamins can contribute to morning sickness and nausea
during pregnancy. Eating six small meals rather than
three large ones helps, as does nibbling on a small dry

snack (whole wheat toast) before getting out of bed in the morning.

- A cup of basil or red raspberry tea, plain or with a little honey, can ease queasiness and help prevent vomiting.
- Two capsules of red raspberry concentrate, taken in the morning, has been found to alleviate nausea, particularly in the first trimester.
- Chewing on a stick of ginger, taking a ginger root capsule, or sipping a cup of ginger tea has helped many a lady-in-waiting overcome unpleasant intestinal unrest.
- Vitamin B complex, (time release), 50 mg., twice daily, can work as a preventive. (Vitamin B_6 has long been used in many commercial antinausea preparations.)

HEARTBURN

Another common pregnancy discomfort, usually due to indigestion caused by an increase or decrease in gastric juices, is heartburn.

- Try potato juice! Potatoes are a great source of alkaline ingredients, which can reduce acidity. Simply grate a potato, strain, and drink the juice for natural relief.
- Drink cold liquids through a straw, to avoid swallowing excess air.
- Peppermint tea can soothe that uncomfortable burning sensation, and relax you as well.
- Avoid fried, spicy, and fatty foods, as well as alcohol, chocolate, coffee, colas, and cigarettes.

CONSTIPATION

Since pregnancy hormones can slow down the digestive system, it needs all the help it can get.

- Drink liquids, and plenty of them! Upon rising, a glass of hot water with a little lemon can work wonders.
- Unprocessed bran and unprocessed wheat germ, 1 tbsp. each, daily. (These work better when moistened. Use milk, juice, or soup according to taste.)
- Licorice tea works well as a mild laxative.

CAUTION: Drinking large amounts may elevate blood pressure.

- Be sure your meals include ample amounts of whole grains, fresh fruits, and raw vegetables. (These create needed bulk.)
- A good supplement regimen would be:
  Acidophilus liquid   1 tbsp., 3 times daily
  Bran tablets   3–9 daily

HEMORRHOIDS

These are torturous swellings of the veins under the lining of the anus and lower rectum—and the scourge of pregnant women. The swellings become more prominent when you strain at stool and can enlarge quite suddenly and fill with blood clots, which can be quite painful and may break down and bleed profusely for several days.

- One tablespoon of unprocessed bran, 3 times daily.
- Vitamin C complex, 1,000 mg., 2–4 times daily (helps keep stool soft and strengthens the walls of the blood vessels)
- Vitamin E, 200–400 IU, 1–3 times daily (helps prevent and dissolve clots)
- Vitamin E oil, applied topically to afflicted area, can reduce discomfort.

- Avoid coffee, chocolate, cocoa, and cola, as these can increase anal itching.
- When lifting objects, stoop instead of bending. This reduces abdominal pressure on hemorrhoidal veins.

WATER RETENTION

- Vitamin B_6, 50–100 mg., taken 3 times daily can act as a natural diuretic.

INSOMNIA

When you're pregnant, you need a proper amount of rest, but learn that this is frequently easier said than done.

- A glass of warm milk at bedtime. (Milk is high in tryptophan, which works as a safe and natural sedative and tranquilizer.)
- Chamomile tea, an old standby that still works.
- Supplements for sleep:

Tryptophan tabs 500–667 mg.	3 tabs, taken ½ hour before bedtime with water or juice (no protein)
Chelated calcium and magnesium	1 tab, 3 times daily
Vitamin B_6	50 mg., ½ hour before bedtime

79. The Right Exercises Right Through

The feeling about exercise during pregnancy has changed drastically over the past several decades. In fact, the phrase "period of confinement" is rarely used nowadays as a synonym for pregnancy. And for good reason.

As long as proper precautions are observed, most doctors are in favor of exercise for pregnant women. Exercise can not only tone you up for labor by strengthening your abdomen, pelvis, pubic muscles, and lower limbs but can also help control and coordinate your breathing as well. Some doctors even feel that you can safely continue your prepregnancy exercises—with the exception of jogging, aerobic dancing, or any involving jumping and bouncing. (Some exercises that are done lying down on your back are also contraindicated because they could force the fetus on top of the placenta and cut off its nutrition and oxygen.)

Nonetheless, there are circumstances when, and individuals for whom, exercise is *not* recommended.

EXERCISE DURING PREGNANCY IS NOT ADVISED IF . . .

- you have a history of miscarriage;
- you have high blood pressure, anemia, diabetes, or any serious health problem;
- you haven't checked with your doctor.

CAUTION: Discontinue any exercise at the first sign of vaginal bleeding, pain, heart palpitations, or shortness of breath. Never overexert yourself!

80. Special Nutrition for First-time Mothers Over Thirty

Perhaps the greatest nutritional difference between mothers over thirty and those under is the former's need for more calcium. Pregnant or not, the older a woman gets, the greater her need for calcium.

Calcium pills are not advised as a replacement for

milk, unless prescribed by a doctor, but if you dislike drinking milk, you can always disguise it in soups, puddings, quiches, and a variety of other dishes. For example:

DANDI COTTAGE SCRAMBLES
(1 serving = approx. 82 mg. calcium)

2 eggs
1 scant tbsp. butter
   or fortified
   margarine

pepper to taste
½ cup cottage cheese
   (2% fat)

Beat eggs. Melt butter in frying pan and pour in eggs. As they begin to set, add cottage cheese and then scramble in pan until done. Add salt and pepper. (One serving)

BANANA BEAUTY
(1 serving = approx. 296 mg. calcium)

2 sliced ripe bananas

¼ cup orange juice
dash of vanilla

2 cups reconstituted
   nonfat dry milk (but
   substitute 1 cup ice
   cubes for each cup
   water)

Put ingredients into blender—adding ice slowly— and blend until thick and creamy. (Two to three servings)

HONEY HEAVEN
(1 serving = approx. 296 mg. calcium)

1 cup skim (or low-fat)
   milk
1 tsp. honey

¾ tsp. vanilla
cinnamon

Warm milk, honey, and vanilla, then pour quickly in blender to froth. Serve and sprinkle with cinnamon. (One serving)

For other calcium-rich foods, see section 36. (Using tahini—which is made from sesame seeds— mixed with yogurt makes a fine dip for raw calcium-rich and low-calorie vegetables, such as broccoli.)

Also be sure to include plenty of foods rich in vitamin B$_6$ and folic acid in your diet, particularly whole grains and vegetables.

SUPPLEMENT SUGGESTIONS

- High-potency multiple vitamin and mineral, A.M. and P.M.
- Multiple chelated minerals (2 tablets should equal 1,000 mg. calcium and 500 mg. magnesium), A.M. and P.M.
- Folic acid, 800 mcg., 3 times daily

CAUTION: The above regimen, and all others in the book, are not prescriptive nor intended as medical advice. Before starting any regimen, check with your doctor or a nutritionally oriented physician (see section 145).

81. Herbs That Work as Pregnancy Supplements

Alfalfa	As a supplement, 3 capsules daily (with meals) can supply a mother-to-be with an assortment of vitamins, ample calcium, and adequate magnesium.
Parsley	Eight sprigs as a garnish or two capsules daily are an excellent source of iron, potassium, and phosphorus, and can help reduce water retention.
Beet Root	A great natural supplier of iron that will not constipate the way regular iron supplements might.

Gotu Kola	Not to be confused with the kola nut, which contains caffeine, a nondesirable for shaping up (see section 130), gotu kola is rich in B vitamins, and supplements of 2–4 capsules daily with meals can help women cope more easily with the stresses of pregnancy and childbirth.
Fenugreek	One cup of fenugreek tea, or two supplemental capsules daily, helps provide strength and elasticity to uterine muscles and tissues. This herb has been found to be especially effective if used during the last six weeks of pregnancy.

82. Herbs To Avoid During Pregnancy and Breast-Feeding

Goldenseal	Very similar to morphine and not advised for pregnant or lactating women.
Valerian	A strong sedative, and not recommended.
Skullcap	Very similar to valerian, and again not recommended.
Senna	A laxative that could be dangerous if taken in the first months of pregnancy by inducing miscarriage.
Buckthorn	Very similar to senna, and equally contraindicated.
Kola nut	Contains caffeine, and not advised. (See section 130.)
Guarana	Contains caffeine, and should be avoided in all its forms.

NOTE: It's advisable to steer clear of all strong and pungent spices, such as capsicum, horseradish, and so on. If you're breast-feeding, be aware that garlic and onions will pass through to the breast milk and might cause colic.

83. Cures for Postpartum Blues

It's not unusual for a woman to experience a letdown after the birth of a baby. Aside from the fatigue of labor, there are hormonal changes in the body that often cause bouts of blues and periods of inexplicable weepiness or mild depression. But these can be combatted by paying special attention to your diet.

- Be sure you're getting enough calcium and calcium-rich foods; also, the proper amount of magnesium. (The combination is a natural depression defeater.) As a supplement, 1,000–1,500 mg. chelated calcium and 500–750 mg. magnesium, daily.
- Vitamins B_1, B_6, and B_{12} can help improve mental attitude substantially. As a supplement, 50–100 mg. of vitamins B_1 and B_6, and 50–100 mcg. of B_{12}, twice daily.
- L-tryptophan, a natural relaxant and antidepressant, can pass rapidly from the stomach to the brain's nerve centers. (Turkey is especially high in this amino acid.) As a supplement, 500–667 mg. once or twice daily, between meals, with water or juice.
- Manganese, present in leafy green vegetables, peas, egg yolks, beets, and whole-grain cereals, has been found by many new mothers to be effective in warding off depression.
- L-phenylalanine is another amino acid and can work in a fashion similar to tryptophan, but unlike L-tryptophan, L-phenylalanine can raise blood pressure. As a supplement, 250–500 mg., once or twice daily, with water or juice. (See "Cautions," section 124.)

NOTE: For a quick reference list of foods containing these nutrients, see section 36.

84. So Long, Stretch Marks

A sudden weight gain for any reason can cause stretch marks, those first reddish and then pearly white lines that just never seem to go away. Well, the truth is that the best way to get rid of them is to nip them in the bud—obviously, easier said than done.

If you are pregnant, a daily application of vitamin E oil really elasticizes that stretching skin, as does cocoa butter. (Gaining weight slowly is the best preventive.) Taking 200–400 IU vitamin E daily, along with 1,000 mg. vitamin C (which is necessary for the formation of collagen) also helps.

But if we're talking after the fact, how about trying one of the all-time great stretch un-markers that was suggested to me by M. J. Saffon in the book *Body Lifts* (Warner Books).

Bring to a boil in an enamel, glass, or stainless-steel pot (not aluminum):

1 4–oz. bar cocoa butter	2 tbsp. apple-cider vinegar
6 tbsp. dried sage	1 qt. water

Cover and simmer for 15 minutes and then let cool to room temperature.

When cool, soak any natural fiber fabric— muslin, cotton, cheesecloth—in the mixture, and then wrap around your body for 20 minutes.

My addition: Rinse in warm shower. Then apply 28,000 IU vitamin E oil topically and leave on overnight. Keep up your supplemental intake of vitamins E and C and watch those stretch marks fade!

85. Nice News for Nursing Mothers

After your baby is born, your body levels of estrogen and progesterone, hormones that promote the growth of fat cells, decrease. This is good news for new mothers who are anxious to regain their figures, because not only are these hormones that promoted water retention and increased appetite on the wane, but they're replaced by a new hormone, prolactin, that promotes the burning of fat to make milk.

While breast-feeding, you can burn an extra 800–1,500 calories a day! But before you take this as a cue to indulge your junk-food fantasies, think twice—for you and your baby. The foods you want now are low-fat dairy products, fresh raw vegetables, whole grains, and lean protein; foods that will help stabilize your metabolism and appetite (allowing you to take off pounds and *keep* them off) while providing you and your infant with optimal nutrition.

86. Be Doubly Careful When You're Feeding Two

As a nursing mother, you are the sole source of your child's food supply, and your milk will be only as nutritious as you make it.

Your daily diet should include the following:

Milk—a quart a day (low-fat, fat-free, whole, evaporated, or skim) in any form; and lots of extra fluids:

Meat, fish, poultry, eggs—at least one serving daily;

Fruits and vegetables—several servings daily, and they should include plenty of leafy dark-green vegetables and fresh vitamin-C-rich fruits;

Whole-grain cereals and breads—three servings to provide ample B vitamins and energy.

A multivitamin-mineral supplement to provide enough

vitamin D to allow you to properly use the calcium in your diet.

CAUTION: *If you're a nursing mother, consult your doctor before taking any medication. Many drugs can enter breast milk—and what's good for you is not necessarily good for your child. (NOTE: The fact that a particular medication does not appear on the following list should in no way be construed that it is harmless to your nursing infant. Always consult your doctor before taking a medicine if you are breast-feeding.)*

DRUGS THAT MAY HARM A NURSING BABY

Amphetamines	Drugs used as central nervous stimulants (CNS) to control weight, narcolepsy, and hyperactivity in children and sometimes teenagers
Atropine	Atropisol—an ophthalmic medication used in the eye to dilate the pupil
Barbiturates	Central nervous system (CNS) depressants used as tranquilizers and sedatives
Belladonna alkaloids and barbiturates	Drugs containing atropine, hyoscyamine, scopolamine, butabarbital, pentobarbital, phenobarbital, or amobarbital used in combination to relieve cramping, spasms of stomach, intestines or bladder

Benzodiazepines	Drugs used as tranquilizers and sedatives, including Librium, Valium, Dalmane, Ativan, Serax, and Verstran, among others
Cascara sagrada	A stimulant laxative
Chloralhydrate	Usually used as a sedative or hypnotic; common brand names are Noctec and Oradrate
Chloramphenicol	Chloromycetin—an antibiotic
Corticosteroids	Anti-inflammatory medications used to relieve symptoms of arthritis, asthma, skin problems, and severe allergies
Cyclophosphamide	Cytoxan—an antineoplastic or anticancer medication
Danthron	A stimulant laxative found in such brands as Dorbane and Modane
Dicumarol	An anticoagulant, or blood thinner
Ergotamine	An antimigraine medication found in brands such as Ergomar and Ergostat
Estrogens	Female hormones often used to regulate menstrual cycle, in birth control pills, after certain types of surgery
Isoniazid	Drug used for tuberculosis
Levodopa	Drug used for the treatment of Parkinson's disease

Lindane	A topical treatment for scabies and lice infections; common brand names are Kwell and Scabene
Lithium carbonate	An antidepressant
Meperidine	A pain-killer; most common brand is Demerol
Meprobamate	A tranquilizer and sedative, found in such name brands as Equanil and Miltown, among others
Methotrexate	An antineoplastic—anticancer—drug
Metronidazole	An anti-infective, usually used for genital-urinary tract infections; most common brand name is Flagyl
Nalidixic acid	A urinary antibacterial; most common brand name is NegGram
Oral contraceptives	Birth control pills containing hormones, estrogens, and/or progestins
Penicillin G sodium	An antibiotic
Phenolphthalein	A stimulant laxative, found in such brands as Ex-Lax and Feen-A-Mint, among others
Phenylbutazone	Drugs used to treat symptoms of certain types of arthritis and joint disease; common brand names are Butazolidin and Azolid

Phenytoin	An anticonvulsant; most common brand is Dilantin
Potassium iodide	An expectorant
Primidone	An anticonvulsant; most common brand is Mysoline
Streptomycin	An antibiotic; has many name brands
Sulfisoxazole	A urinary antibacterial; common name brand is Gantrisin
Tetracycline	An antibiotic; has many name brands
Thiazides	A diuretic used often to treat high blood pressure
Valproic acid	An anticonvulsant; common brand name is Depakene
Warfarin	An anticoagulant; common name brands are Coumadin and Panwarfarin, among others

87. Any Questions About Chapter IV?

Do you know of any natural treatments to ease childbirth?

According to several medical studies and quite a few mothers I've met, red raspberry leaf tea eases and speeds up labor.

Squeeze the juice of an orange into a cup of strong, red raspberry leaf tea (one ounce of dried leaves steeped in 20 ounces of boiling water will make more than a day's supply). Drink one to three cups, or about a pint daily, during the last month of pregnancy.

I'm a vegetarian and planning to nurse my baby. Some of my friends say that I won't be giving the baby proper nutrition. Is this true?

Not at all, as long as you get enough nutrients from vegetarian sources. (See below.) In fact, it's been shown that vegetarian mothers have considerably less pollutant chemicals in their breast milk than their meat-eating sisters. This has been attributed to the fact that many chemicals enter the body as a contaminant of animal fat and are then stored in human fat.

What I'd advise is making sure that your daily intake of protein, calcium, vitamins B_2, B_{12}, D, iron, and zinc is sufficient. Your best sources would be:

For protein:	Legumes combined with grains, nuts, or seeds; or a combination of any plant food with dairy products or eggs
For calcium:	Aside from dairy products, you can get a good supply from fortified soy milk, legumes, dark-green leafy vegetables, as well as nuts and seeds.
For vitamins B_2, B_{12}:	Whole grains, brewer's yeast, dark-green leafy vegetables, dairy products, and supplements (A balanced B complex with at least 3 mcg. of vitamin B_{12}, taken 1–3 times daily is recommended.)
For vitamin D:	Fortified soy or regular milk, and a good multivitamin (which your doctor has probably advised) will fill the bill.
For iron:	Dark-green leafy vegetables, torula yeast, whole grains, dried fruits Combining citrus fruits with iron-rich foods will help you get the most of your iron.

For zinc: Wheat germ, whole grains, eggs, cheese, legumes, and nuts

My friend, who's pregnant, has been using lecithin to control her weight gain. Is this safe?

I would *not* advise taking it during pregnancy. Though lecithin is a natural fat emulsifier found in eggs, nuts, soybeans, and liver— among other natural foods—and has been used safely with kelp, vinegar, and vitamin B₆ as a diet aid for years, recent studies on animals done by Dr. Joanne Bell, of the department of pharmacology at Duke University Medical Center in Durham, North Carolina, have shown that lecithin when given to pregnant females *can* cause birth defects.

Altering eating habits, and not using diet aids, is the *only* safe way to control weight during pregnancy! Keep in mind that if a mother is inadequately nourished, it can affect fetal growth, which is why doctors no longer restrict weight gain to twenty pounds, but are more in favor of a twenty-eight to thirty-pound gain.

Is it safe to use hair dyes during pregnancy?

Though blondes—and I suspect brunettes and redheads, too—have more fun, they should be aware that hair dyes are absorbed by the scalp, and the chemicals in those dyes can be transmitted to the fetus. This is not to say that they will cause congenital problems in the fetus, but the possibility exists and should not be ignored.

My advice is, if you want to color your hair during pregnancy, ask your doctor about the ingredients in the specific product you are using.

I realize that no food additives are good for you, but I'm wondering if there are any that you know of that should be avoided by pregnant women in particular?

Avoid all those that have been implicated as possible carcinogens, particularly:

- Saccharin
- Cyclamates
- Sodium nitrite and sodium nitrate (used in most luncheon meats, hot dogs, and smoked or cured commercial products)
- Artificial coloring (especially citrus Red No. 2, Orange B, Red No. 3, Red No. 40, and Yellow No. 5)
- BHT (butylated hydroxytoluene)

I'd also recommend avoiding as many artificial flavorings as possible, as well as quinine (which flavors tonic water and bitter lemon), as this has been implicated in causing birth defects; sulfur dioxide and sodium bisulfite (which can destroy vitamin B_1); MSG (monosodium glutamate); BHA (butylated hydroxyanisole); phosphoric acid and phosphates (which can cause dietary imbalances and have recently been implicated as a factor in the spreading of osteoporosis).

How dangerous, really, are coffee and alcohol for pregnant women? My mother drank coffee and alcohol during her pregnancy and had no problems.

Your mother was lucky; other pregnant women might not be. Animal studies have shown that large amounts of caffeine (which coffee, cocoa, chocolate, cola, and many medications contain) may cause birth defects. And alcohol, even in moderate amounts (a couple of highballs a night), can result in low infant birth weight, as well as cause physical or behavioral abnormalities in the child.

Coffee substitutes, such as caffeine-free Postum, Pero, or Kafix, are easily available. As for alcohol, I'd advise staying away from it completely. (A wine glass filled with sparkling salt-free seltzer and a wedge of lemon or lime can be psychologically and socially satisfying—and safe.) I'd also recommend checking the labels of any medication you're taking to be sure they don't contain either of these two drugs.

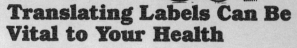

Translating Labels Can Be Vital to Your Health

WHAT THE LABEL SAYS	TRANSLATION
"Low-calorie"	Can have 40 calories a serving
"Hi-energy"	High calorie
"Measurable amounts of important nutrients needed to maintain good health"	Not necessarily more than 2 percent of the RDA for those nutrients
"Natural"	Not defined by the Federal Trade Commission and therefore is often wildly deceptive
"Made with real honey"	Usually contains more real granulated sugar, brown sugar, and high-fructose corn syrup
"No preservatives"	Can still contain other chemical additives
"Low sodium"	Can contain 140 mg. per serving
"No cholesterol"	Not necessarily low in fat
"Naturally flavored"	The *flavor* is derived from a natural product, and that's usually all
"Enriched wheat flour"	Essentially, white flour

Think about it . . .

V.

Looking Good

88. Total Skin Shape-up

For really sensational-looking skin, you have to work from the inside out. The right nutrients are a necessity. They feed the nerves, tissues, and blood vessels, act as cleansing agents, and all in all keep your epidermis looking vital, smooth, and healthy. No cosmetic in the world can substitute for good nutrition!

NEEDED NUTRIENTS: (For a list of foods containing these nutrients, see section 36.)

VITAMIN A

Preserves the skin's elasticity and smoothness, helps delay wrinkles, aids in growth and repair of tissues, builds resistance to skin infections and blemishes. Too little vitamin A in your diet can result in flaky, itchy, or goose-bumped skin. As a supplement: Use the dry form. 25,000 IU, twice daily, A.M. and P.M., for five days a week and then stop for two.

VITAMIN C

Vital for the production of collagen, which strengthens connective tissue, promotes healing of wounds, bruises, and scar tissue, aids in the prevention of capillary breakage ("spider lines"), protects skin from chemical pollutants, helps fight acne and other infections by stimulating the production of white blood cells.

As a supplement: Rose hips vitamin C, 1,000 mg. (with bioflavonoids), three times daily. (Take one with each meal and then at bedtime.)

VITAMIN E

Maintains and preserves cell membranes, improves circulation in tiny capillaries on the face, aids in healing, and works with vitamin C to keep blood vessels healthy and less subject to blemishes, also keeps skin younger-looking by retarding cell aging.

As a supplement: Use the dry form, 200–400 IU, one to three times daily. Take after meals.

(Vitamin E oil, 28,000 IU, can be applied externally for healing burns, abrasions, and scar tissue.)

VITAMIN B COMPLEX

Essential for smooth and unblemished skin; vitamins B_2 and B_6 help reduce oiliness and the formation of blackheads.

As a supplement: Vitamin B complex, 100 mg. (time release), one daily, taken after any meal.

CHOLINE AND INOSITOL

These help emulsify cholesterol and eliminate fatty deposits or bumps under the skin. They also act as cleansing agents by helping to purify the kidneys.

As a supplement: 1,000 mg., daily, taken after a large meal. (Lecithin granules, 2 tsp., daily, can be substituted for choline and inositol tabs.)

ZINC

Aids in growth and repair of injured tissues, and promotes in healing of wounds and skin infections.

As a supplement: Chelated zinc, 15–50 mg., daily.

CYSTEINE

Helps keep skin soft and supple, aids in inhibiting the aging process of skin and the formation of wrinkles.

As a supplement: 1 gram daily, between meals, with juice or water (no protein). For best results, take 3 times as much Vitamin C as cysteine.

ACIDOPHILUS

Aids in the prevention of skin eruptions caused by unfriendly bacteria in the system.

As a supplement: 3 tbsp., daily. Take 1 tbsp. —or 2 capsules—after each meal.

CHLOROPHYLL

A wound-healer and a prime stimulant for the growth of new tissue; also helps prevent bacterial contamination of skin.

As a supplement: 3 tsp. or nine tablets, daily. Take 1 tsp.—or three tabs—after each meal.

MUST MINERALS

Calcium is important for soft smooth skin tissue; copper for skin color; iron to improve pale or lifeless skin; potassium for dry skin and acne; zinc for external and internal wound-healing.

As a supplement: If your eating habits are erratic and you're not getting sufficient amounts of these minerals, I'd recommend two multiple chelated mineral tablets daily, after a large meal, or one in A.M. and P.M.

Also, for general all-over skin tone and health, I'd recommend a multiple-vitamin and mineral complex be taken daily. And don't forget about exercise! Circulation-building aerobics bring blood and more nutrients to the skin.

89. Know Your Skin's Enemies

No matter how terrific your skin might be, it has enemies. And they are ruthless. By being aware of who the bad guys are and what they can do, you will help to protect your skin from unnecessary harm.

THE BAD GUYS	WHAT THEY CAN DO	HOW TO FIGHT BACK
Sunlight	Ultraviolet radiation penetrates the skin and damages the collagen that supports it as well as the blood vessels that supply its nourishment; dries, wrinkles, and ages skin.	Use a sunscreen. PABA ointment, or any with a sun-protecting factor (SPF) of 15 or higher. Be sure you're getting enough vitamins A, C, E, and zinc.
Alcohol	Dehydrates the skin, dilates blood vessels, and contributes to broken capillaries, interferes with proper nutrient metabolism.	Cut down on alcohol consumption. Up your intake of vitamins E, A, and C. Apply vitamin E oil, 28,000 IU, to your skin daily.
Cigarette smoking	Damages collagen, depletes vitamin C (necessary for collagen), causes wrinkles, blood vessel constriction, and sallow skin.	Stop smoking! Increase your intake of vitamin C (1,000 mg. daily) and take an equal amount of pantothenic acid.
Caffeine	Dehydrates skin; depletes B vitamins, potassium, and zinc; inhibits calcium and iron assimilation.	Keep away from coffee, chocolate, tea, cocoa, and cola beverages; take B complex supplement, 100 mg. and zinc, 15–50 mg., daily. Cover

The Bad Guys	What They Can Do	How To Fight Back
		your bases with a good high-potency multivitamin and mineral supplement daily.
Diuretics	Dehydrate skin; deplete 8 vitamins, potassium, magnesium, and zinc.	Supplement diet with a complete multiple B complex and multiple mineral; moisten skin and apply a thin film of Crisco, massage gently and leave on overnight.
Crash diets	When weight is lost too quickly, the skin loses elasticity.	Diet sensibly and lose weight at the rate of no more than two pounds a week; up your intake of foods rich in vitamins A, C, and E.
Stress	Can cause wrinkles; releases aging chemicals in the body; interferes with sleep and proper diet.	Increase vitamin-B-rich foods in diet; take vitamin B complex, 100 mg., 1–3 times daily, along with L-tryptophan, 500–667 mg., 1–3 times daily (with water or juice— no pro-

tein), and chelated calcium and magnesium, 3 tabs, 3 times daily.

Use protective windscreen (PABA ointment, or any with an SPF of 15 or higher). Be sure you're getting enough vitamins A, C, E, and zinc. Moisturize skin with vitamin E oil daily.

Dehydrates and chaps skin.

Cold air and wind

90. Disaster Drugs for Your Skin

There are indeed times when drugs can work miracles, but very often they can wreak havoc on your skin. Unfortunately, most doctors never mention the cosmetic side effects a particular medication might have, which is why I've compiled the following list. It is not all-inclusive, but should let you know that if a dermatological side effect does occur because of the medication you're taking, you can at least ask your doctor about the possibility of taking an alternative drug.

DRUG	POSSIBLE COSMETIC SIDE EFFECT
Amytal	Skin rash, swollen eyelids, itchy skin
Butisol	Acne, pimples
Dalmane	Rash, flushes
Dexamyl	Itchy skin, swollen patches
Dexedrine	Itchy skin, swollen patches
Equanil	Welts, rash, dermatitis
Librium	Pimples
Miltown	Welts, flaking skin, itching
Nembutal	Rash
Phenobarbital	Rash, itchy skin, swollen eyelids
Placidyl	Itchy skin, swollen patches
Talwin	Facial swelling, rash, skin peeling
Tetracycline	Sunburn
Thorazine	Peeling skin, jaundice, welts, swelling
Tofranil	Itchy skin, rash, jaundice
Tuinal	Can aggravate existing skin conditions
Valium	Jaundice, rash, swollen patches

91. Treating Psoriasis Without Steroids

Psoriasis, a disease characterized by red patches on the skin, often covered with silvery scales, is more a cosmetically than physically debilitating disease. Nonetheless, it's a serious problem for those who suffer from it—and even more serious for those who take prescription steroids to alleviate it.

Steroidal therapy can cause major nutrient losses of calcium and phosphorus, contribute to adrenal exhaustion, weaken the immune system, and promote depression, among other undesirable side effects. But there are alternatives, and I'd recommend trying them before resorting to prescription drugs.

Daily topical applications of vitamins A and D oils have improved the skin condition of psoriasis sufferers dramatically; as has increased protein intake and the following supplement regimen:

- A high-potency multiple vitamin with chelated minerals, A.M. and P.M.
- Vitamin C, 1,000 mg., with bioflavonoids, rutin, hesperidin, and rose hips, 2–4 times daily.
- High-potency chelated multiple mineral tablet, A.M. and P.M.
- Vitamin A (water soluble), 10,000 IU, 3 times daily for 5 days a week.
- Vitamin B complex, 100 mg. (time release), A.M. and P.M.
- Vitamin E (dry form), 100–400 IU, 3 times daily
- Lecithin capsules, 1,200 mg., three, 3 times daily

92. Acne: It's Not Just Kid Stuff

Acne is a disease, and not just a phase teenagers go through. In fact, it's on the rise in women over twenty-one.

Acne sufferers usually have a genetic proclivity for the disease, a structural defect in the skin that makes pores function differently. But there are certain factors that do aggravate acne, and you should know them.

ACNE ACTIVATORS

STRESS: It can be emotional or physical, negative or positive, even brought on by drinking too much coffee.

ULTRAVIOLET LIGHT: Too much sun can irritate the skin and worsen the condition.

MANY BIRTH CONTROL PILLS: Also other medications (see section 90).

CERTAIN COSMETICS: For a list of acne-irritating ingredients contained in commonly sold cosmetics, send a self-addressed envelope to the ACNE Research Institute, 1587 Monrovia, Newport Beach, CA 92663.

OILS OR CHEMICALS: Contact can be direct or as indirect as working in a garage or at a greasy grill.

ABRASIVE SCRUBS: Or too much rubbing of affected skin. Keep skin clean, but overdoing washing can aggravate acne conditions.

IODINE, IODIZED SALT: Eliminate all salted and processed foods, which are usually high in salt that has been iodized and can worsen acne.

HELPFUL SUPPLEMENTS

- Multiple vitamin with minerals (but *low* in iodine), 1 daily
- Vitamin E (dry form), 400 IU, 1–2 daily
- Vitamin A, 25,000 IU (water soluble), 1–2 daily, 5 days a week (stop for two)
- Zinc, chelated, 15–50 mg., 3 times daily with meals
- Acidophilus liquid, 1–2 tbsp., 3 times daily, or 3–6 capsules, 3 times daily

93. Solving Special Skin Problems for Men

Let's face it, shaving your face daily or every other day takes its toll on the skin, and often leaves a man's face more in need of conditioning than a woman's. Additionally, using after-shave lotions that are high in alcohol only worsens the problem by drying out the skin even more.

> Beware of the tingle! An after-shave lotion that makes your face tingle is doing more damage than good.

If your face looks red or blotchy after shaving, your skin is more sensitive than you think and needs help. Before shaving, wash your face with a *mild* soap, then be sure to leave your shaving cream on for at least one minute to promote maximum beard softening. After shaving, avoid lotions that have more than 20 percent alcohol. (Beware of the tingle! Most after-shaves have an 80 to 90 percent alcohol content that can really dry and irritate your skin.)

If you use an electric razor, you want to remove as much water as you can from the skin's surface. There are special powders available, but a light dusting of plain talc will work as well.

To prevent or clear up facial rashes and redness, men would be well advised to increase the vitamin-B-rich foods in their diets (see section 36). If the face becomes irritated, a topical application of vitamin E oil will soothe and speed healing.

A good supplement program would be:

- High-potency multiple vitamin, 1 daily
- Vitamin E (dry form), 200–400 IU, 1–2 times daily
- Vitamin A (dry form), 10,000 IU, 1–2 times daily, for 5 days a week

- Chelated zinc, 15–50 mg., 3 times daily with food
- Acidophilus liquid, 3 times daily, or 3–6 capsules, 3 times daily

94. Reducing Wrinkles Without Surgery

> Even leaning your cheek on your hand too often can cause wrinkles.

For openers: Moisturize! Moisturization is essential to maintaining young-looking skin and staving off wrinkles. The best time to do it is *after* bathing or washing. You want the skin to absorb the water and then seal it in with oil or some other lubricant.

Most dermatologists recommend not adding bath oil to your tub immediately, but waiting until you've soaked for at least fifteen minutes, if you want your skin to benefit.

Supplements of vitamin C, 1,000 mg., and pantothenic acid, 1,000 mg., daily can help stave off wrinkles.

Keeping your body supplied with vitamin C will keep collagen—which is responsible for the stability and strength of practically all bodily tissues, including the skin—strong and elastic. Vitamins A, B complex, fatty acids, and minerals are also important.

To reduce and prevent wrinkles, avoid your skin's enemies (see section 89) and try not to stretch your facial skin by either gaining and losing weight rapidly, frowning or squinting, or even leaning your cheek on your hand too often.

95. The Collagen Controversy

The collagen that's found in cosmetics and used in injections to correct wrinkles is a natural protein that is derived from the skin of cows and has the same amino acid makeup as human collagen.

Though it has FDA approval for use as a wrinkle treatment, you should be aware that certain people can be allergic to it. If you are going to have a doctor treat your skin with collagen injections, be sure that you are given tests for an allergic reaction beforehand.

96. How To Put Your Best Face Forward

To soap or not to soap is often the question. The answer is that soap and nonsoap cleansers are basically designed to do the same thing—remove dirt, oil, sweat; remove dead skin and unclog pores. Nonsoap cleansers are usually made from synthetic detergent compounds such as petroleum-based derivatives, but these have been found to work better in areas where there is hard water.

EASY-TO-FOLLOW WASHING INSTRUCTIONS

- Use a soap that rinses off your skin easily (this is less likely to cause irritation).
- If using a washcloth, make sure it's soft, and already dampened. (A cloth can help slough off dead skin cells.)
- Use warm and not hot water. (Hot water expands blood vessels and can aggravate skin irritations.)
- Wash gently. (Rubbing soap into the face can clog pores.)
- Rinse thoroughly.
- Avoid perfumed or deodorant soaps for facial use. (If you have been using a topical antibiotic for a skin condition, the ingredients in a deodorant soap could interfere with the antibiotic action.)
- To protect dry skin, or prevent skin from unnecessary

aging, use a superfatted soap (Dove, Basis, Alpha Keri, and so on) that will leave an invisible film of oil on and help prevent moisture loss.

• To restore a protective acid mantle to your skin, after washing finish with a splash of ordinary vinegar (a weak acid). It can be a skin rejuvenator.

97. Keeping Your Crowning Glory in Royal Shape

Hair contains all the vitamins and minerals and other nutrients the body needs for health, and is about 97 percent protein. Because of this, an inadequate diet will not only affect the way you feel but also the condition of your hair as well. And there are no shampoos or conditioners that will compensate for inadequate nutrition. Unlike skin, hair cannot repair itself—but you *can* get new, healthier hair to grow!

NEEDED NUTRIENTS

VITAMIN B COMPLEX (*choline, inositol, biotin, pantothenic acid, folic acid, PABA*)

> All members of the B complex family of vitamins are essential for hair replacement and growth. (A severe folic acid deficiency could cause baldness.) Pantothenic acid and PABA also retard hair loss and have in some cases reversed the premature graying of hair and restored it to natural color.
>
> *As a supplement:* Vitamin B complex, 100 mg. (time release), 1–3 daily

CYSTEINE

> This amino acid comprises approximately 10–14 percent of the hair shaft, the portion above the surface of the skin. It contributes to hair luster.

As a supplement: 1 gram daily, taken between meals with water or juice. (Taking vitamin C, 1,000 mg., 3 times daily will make the cysteine work more effectively.)

VITAMIN A
Keeps hair shiny and works in conjunction with B vitamins.
As a supplement: 10,000 IU, 1–2 times daily, 5 days a week

MULTIPLE CHELATED MINERALS
These help prevent hair from falling out.
As a supplement: 1 daily with breakfast

MULTIPLE VITAMIN AND MINERAL COMPLEX
This is essential for the general health of your hair. In combination with other supplements, it helps fight pollution that can adversely affect your hair's condition.
As a supplement: 1 daily after any meal
And don't forget exercise and sleep!

98. How To Thicken Thin Hair
Hair is shed and regrown daily. Heredity plays a major role in whether your lost hairs are going to be readily replaced, but so does handling and diet.
• Avoid rough scalp massages and towel drying, perming and hot blow-drying (these weaken the hair shaft).
• Never set hair dryer on hot (use medium setting) and hold blower at least 6 inches from hair.
• Use a wide-tooth comb to untangle hair and minimize brushing.
• Be sure you're getting enough biotin-rich foods in your diet (see section 36).

- After shampooing, rub a *few* drops of jojoba oil into your hair and scalp. DO NOT rinse. (If your hair is oily, DO rinse.)
- Supplement your diet with:

> Stress B complex (with biotin), 100 mg., twice daily
>
> Choline and inositol, 1,000 mg. of each, daily
>
> A multiple mineral formula with 1,000 mg. calcium and 500 mg. magnesium, daily
>
> Cysteine, 1,000 mg., daily
>
> Vitamin C, 3,000 mg., daily

99. If You're Gray and Don't Like It That Way

Instead of trying to wash away those gray hairs, why not see if some extra B vitamins can't do the trick. Increase your intake of foods rich in pantothenic, folic, and para-aminobenzoic acids (PABA) and see what happens. These are all available as individual supplements, or in a good B complex tablet, which should be taken one to three times daily.

100. The Eyes Have It—If You Eat Right

What you see might be what you get, but what you eat can also affect what and how you see. Nutrition, believe it or not, plays a major role in affecting eyesight.

EYE-OPENING FACTS

- Diets composed of too many processed foods, high in refined carbohydrates and sugar, can contribute to vision problems.

- Nearsightedness and the amount of refined carbohydrates in the diet have been found to be virtually directly proportional.
- Sedative drugs (tranquilizers, sleeping pills) can interfere with nutrient function and affect eyesight adversely.
- Supplements of vitamin B_2 can help alleviate dry or itchy eyes.
- Insufficient intake of vitamin A (or vitamin-A-rich foods) is a contributing factor to night blindness.
- Caffeine can adversely affect eye focus, especially at close range.
- Diets low in zinc prevent the proper release and metabolism of vitamin A, which could contribute to night blindness and other visual problems.

101. Clearing Up Eye Problems Through Nutrition

VITAMIN A

Bugs Bunny was right! Carrots can help, and so can other vitamin-A-rich foods. (See section 36.) This vitamin is the most important vision vitamin. It's necessary for clearness of eye tissues, especially the cornea or front surface of the eye. It prevents eye ulcers and is needed for the production of rhodopsin, a substance that allows us to "recover" our vision after our eyes have been exposed to bright lights.

SPOT QUIZ: *Stare at a bright light for about ten seconds. Then try to read something in large type. If it takes you more than a minute to see again, you might have a vitamin-A deficiency.*

(Dry, inflamed, or light-sensitive eyes can also indicate a vitamin-A deficiency.)

RECOMMENDED SUPPLEMENT: 10,000–25,000 IU, daily (for adults), 5 days a week

ZINC

This mineral is necessary for the proper metabolism and release of vitamin A. If you haven't a sufficient supply of zinc, vitamin A cannot be properly used by the retina and night blindness can occur, as well as dry, itchy eyes.

RECOMMENDED SUPPLEMENT: 15–50 mg. (chelated form), daily

VITAMIN C

This is useful in the treatment (*not cure*) of glaucoma, a disease that *must* be supervised by a physician. As a supplement, though, it has been found to reduce or at least mitigate the effects of increased intraocular (within the eyeball) pressure.

RECOMMENDED SUPPLEMENT: For glaucoma victims (*who must check with physician to be sure it's not contraindicated because of other medications they might be taking*), 1,000 mg., 3 times daily

B COMPLEX VITAMINS

These antistress vitamins are more important to vision than most people realize. They can help prevent eye-muscle paralysis, double vision, night blindness, skin disorders of the lids and skin around the eye, cataracts, and other eye ailments. They're also essential for counteracting the vitamin-depleting effects of refined carbohydrates.

RECOMMENDED SUPPLEMENT: B complex, 100 mg., 1–3 times daily

CALCIUM

Helps in the maintenance of lens transparency in the eye and can aid in the prevention of the development of senile cataracts.

RECOMMENDED SUPPLEMENT: A high-potency multivitamin and mineral tablet that has 1,000 mg. calcium, 500 mg. magnesium, and at least 200 IU of vitamin E, 1–2 times daily

102. Contact Lens Contraindications

There's more to getting contact lenses than getting a good deal. Most optometrists fail to mention that there can be adverse interactions between certain drugs and your contact lenses.

The following drugs can affect contact lenses:

- Insulin
- Diazepam (Valium)
- Nitroglycerin (Nitro-bid)
- Isosorbide dinitrate (Isordil, Sorbitrate)
- Hydralazine hydrochloride (Apresoline, Ser-Ap-Es)
- Warfarin sodium (Coumadin, Panwarfin)
- Rifampin (Rifadin) *Note:* This medication can cause orange discoloration of soft contact lenses, and also cause tears to turn a reddish brown. (It will not discolor hard contact lenses.)

Eyedrop medications such as epinephrine hydrochloride 2% and epinephryl borate 1% can discolor soft contact lenses also.

103. Nifty Nails Can Be a Snap

Looking good right down to your fingertips can be a snap once you realize that the essential ingredient for nifty nails is protein.

A diet with insufficient protein can slow nail growth, as can lack of exercise *and* cold weather.

If you've tried eating gelatin for more beautiful nails and have been disappointed with the results, it's most likely because gelatin alone does not contain all the necessary amino acids (it's an incomplete protein) and must be combined with a complete protein such as milk or bouillon to be effective. In fact, taken alone, gelatin can work against nail growth because of the amino acid imbalance.

All cells in your body require every nutrient to function properly, but certain tissues show deficiencies sooner than others. If you are deficient in vitamins A, C, or zinc, for instance, your nails are most likely to be among the first to reflect this condition.

SUPPLEMENTS FOR SUPER NAILS

- Multiple vitamin with 10,000 IU vitamin A
  Take one or two daily after any meal to promote health and growth of nails.
- Stress B complex with C
  Take one or two with or after meals to help build resistance to fungus infections and to promote nail growth (can also help prevent nail-biting by reducing stress levels).

- Vitamin E (dry form) 200–400 IU
  Take 1–2 times daily for proper utilization of vitamin D and to promote nail growth.
- Multiple chelated mineral
  Take after meals 1–2 times daily. (Iron will help strengthen brittle nails and zinc can help eliminate those white spots.)
- Silica
  This is an organic herb that is changed by the body into readily available organic calcium and can nourish nails. Take 3–6 tablets daily, with meals. Decrease dosage once nails become firm and hard.

TIPS

- *To help soft and splitting nails, avoid putting hands in hot water and keep them away from detergents.*
- *You can stimulate circulation and activate cell growth in slow-growing nails by thrumming them gently on a firm surface, then stretching fingers out and closing into fists several times.*
- *Avoiding polish for a while and painting nails with plain apple cider vinegar have been known to strengthen weak nails.*

NOTE: Little or no growth of nails could indicate a thyroid problem. If supplements don't seem to work, check with a nutritionally oriented doctor. (See section 145.)

104. Easy Steps to Fabulous Feet

Just because they're at the bottom doesn't mean you should ignore them. Uncared for feet, aside from being unattractive and making you look and feel older, can contribute to fatigue, backache, muscle strain, and tension.

1. Keeping away calluses

   Mix 1 tsp. chamomile, 1 tbsp. lemon juice, and 1 clove of garlic (chopped). Rub this onto your calluses and then cover feet for 1–5 minutes with plastic bags. Rinse with warm (not hot) water and then rub calluses with a pumice stone or soft brush. (Regular pumicing after baths or showers can prevent calluses and corns from forming. And so do well-fitting shoes.)

2. Saying bye-bye to bunions

   These painful bumps, usually on the joint of the big toe, are most often caused by tight, ill-fitting shoes, though they can be genetically inherited. Temporary relief can be provided by wearing pads that protect the bunion from friction and by avoiding constricting footwear. Also, since bunions are a form of bursitis, foods rich in vitamins B_{12} (beneficial to cells in bone marrow) and E (helpful in bursitis treatment) are advised. (See section 36.) Supplements of vitamin A, 10,000 IU, daily, and vitamin C, 1,000 mg., daily, should be included in the regimen if there is infection.

3. Tuning up tired feet

   Whenever sitting, rotate ankles, clockwise and then counterclockwise; great for circulation. Also, try a quickie foot massage by putting some dried beans into a pair of flat shoes and walking around in them. Picking up pencils with your toes (or at least attempting to) gives small foot muscles a fine workout. To ease foot strain after a long day, wiggle feet under a stream of hot tub water for several seconds, then do the same under cold. Switch from hot to cold several times. Moisturize your feet afterward by combining an ounce of cocoa butter with an ounce of wheat germ oil and rubbing the mixture over your feet with a wet washcloth.

4. Preventing foot problems

   When purchasing new shoes, always do so at the end

of the day. Your feet can swell as much as 10 percent between morning and late afternoon.

105. Brighten That Smile

Few things are more important to good looks than a great smile, and keeping your teeth, gums, and mouth in fit condition are among the most important prerequisites.

To mention that proper nutrition is essential is, in every way, saying a mouthful. In fact, problems that occur in the mouth are usually a fairly good indicator of a person's general health.

Studies done at the National Institute of Dental Research in Bethesda, Maryland, seem to indicate that many people who have gum disease also suffer from diabetes, heart disease, arthritis, and cataracts, and frequently have the same or very similar dietary deficiencies.

But deficiencies can be rectified, especially if you have regular checkups by a good oral mechanic—a nutritionally oriented dentist (see section 145).

In the meantime, you might be able to alleviate a lot of problems by increasing your intake of high-fiber foods—which require circulation-enhancing chemicals—and by being aware of telltale symptoms and their nutritional remedies.

MINDELL'S MOUTH SHAPE-UP

SYMPTOM	REMEDY
Tooth decay	Keep intake of refined sugars to an absolute minimum and increase the amount of fresh vegetables in your diet. (Have at least 2 green

SYMPTOM	REMEDY
	vegetables with lunch and dinner.) Also, if you can't brush after meals, chew a piece of aged cheese— cheddar or Swiss. Cheese can slow down decay caused by sugar.
Periodontal problems	Increase calcium-rich foods in your diet (see section 36). Try to have at least 3 servings of dark-green leafy vegetables daily. Be sure you're getting adequate amounts of vitamins A, C, E, and zinc, too. A high-potency multiple vitamin with chelated minerals, taken twice daily with meals, would be good insurance.
Bleeding gums	Supplement your diet with vitamin C complex, 1,000 mg., 3 times daily. Since stress can contribute to this condition, a vitamin B complex, 50–100 mg. would be advisable, 1–3 times daily. Rinsing the mouth with comfrey tea has also been found to help.
Canker sores	Increase intake of foods rich in folic acid, iron, niacin, and vitamin B_{12}. (See section 36.) Take a high-potency multiple vitamin with chelated minerals A.M. and P.M. Also, lysine, 500 mg.–1 g., 3 times daily, between meals, with water or juice. When the sores are painful, it's wise to keep away from tobacco; salty, tart, or

Symptom	Remedy
	rough-textured foods; as well as acidic beverages.
Stinging or burning gums (often caused by dentures)	Increase protein intake in diet and double up on fruits and vegetables. Supplement diet with vitamin C, 1,000 mg., 1–2 times daily. Rinse mouth twice daily with comfrey tea.
Thin tooth enamel	Avoid drinking soft water. Supplement diet with a high-potency chelated multiple mineral, A.M. and P.M.

106. What Beauty Experts Don't Tell You About Natural Cosmetics—The Ingredients!

Just because a cosmetic is advertised as "natural" doesn't mean it can't have an adverse effect on you. Allergies to natural substances are very common, which is why I always stress reading labels.

Aloe vera gel, for instance, is an excellent moisturizer and is included in numerous cosmetics. Nonetheless, there are some people who are allergic to it. Knowing whether a product does or does not contain aloe gel, or some derivative of the leaves of the aloe vera plant, could—for those individuals—mean the difference between acquiring a beauty aid or requiring first aid.

Even if you don't know that you're allergic to a particular substance, becoming aware of the ingredients in a cosmetic that doesn't agree with your skin can at least help you in detecting the offending culprit when you find a product with which your skin *is* compatible.

Additionally, knowing what a particular cosmetic contains will make *you*—not the manufacturer or advertiser—the judge of whether it's right for your individual needs. The following list of common cosmetic ingredients has been compiled for that purpose.

Allantoin—an active element of comfrey plant roots; to stimulate formation of healthy cells and relieve skin irritation.

Almond meal—a gentle abrasive powder from ground blanched almonds.

Almond oil—a moisturizer made from crushed almonds.

Aloe vera—a skin softener made from the leaves of the aloe vera plant.

Amyl Dimethyl PABA—a sunscreening agent from PABA, a B-complex factor.

Annatto—a vegetable color obtained from the seeds of a tropical plant.

Apricot oil—a light emollient made from apricot kernels.

Avocado oil—a vegetable oil obtained from avocados.

Azulene—an anti-inflammatory oil made from chamomile flowers.

Beeswax—a purified wax of honeycomb; an emulsifier and thickener.

Camphor—an antibacterial derived from the camphor tree.

Candelilla wax—a hard vegetable wax derived from the candelilla plant and used in lipsticks.

Caprylic/Capric triglyceride—an emollient obtained from coconut oil.

Carnauba wax—derived from palm tree leaves and used in lipsticks.

Carrageenin—a natural thickening agent from dried Irish moss.

Castor oil—an emollient derived from the castor bean.

Cellulose gum—an emulsifier derived from cellulose in wood pulp.

Cetyl alcohol—a solid alcohol that's distilled from plants and vegetables, mostly used as an emollient, stabilizer, or thickener.

Cetyl palmitate—a component of palm and coconut oils.

Chlorophyll—a natural coloring agent and deodorizer derived from plants.

Cholesterin—a lubricant derived from lanolin; cholesterol, but not to be confused with ingested cholesterol.

Cinoxate—a sunscreen derived from cinnamon.

Citric acid—a natural organic acid found widely in citrus plants.

Cocamide DEA—a thickener obtained from coconut oil.

Coconut oil—obtained by pressing the kernels of the seeds of the coconut palm.

Collagen—a protein usually derived from animal connective tissue.

Decyl oleate—obtained from tallow or coconut oil.

Disodium monolaneth-5-sulfosuccinate—obtained from lanolin and used to improve the texture of hair.

Eucalyptus oil—an antiseptic liquid derived from leaves of the eucalyptus tree.

Fragrance—oils obtained from flowers, grasses, roots, and stems that give off a pleasant or agreeable odor.

Glycerin—a humectant and emollient made from vegetable or animal fats and oils.

Glycols—a combination of glycerin and alcohol that is used as a humectant.

Glyceryl stearate—an organic emulsifier obtained from glycerin.

Goat milk whey—protein-rich whey obtained from goat's milk.

Hydrogenated castor oil—a waxy material obtained from castor oil.

Hydroxyethylcellulose—derived from plants or wood pulp; adds thickness to cosmetics.

Imidazolidinyl urea—a preservative derived naturally as a product of protein metabolism (hydrolysis).

Isopropyl palmitate—derived from palmitic acid in coconut oil.

Lanolin—an emollient derived from sheep wool; a natural emulsifier capable of holding water to the skin.

Lanolin alcohol—a constituent of lanolin that performs as an emollient and emulsifier.

Laureth-3—an organic material obtained from coconut and palm oils.

Menthol—derived from mint oils; a natural cooling, anti-irritant.

Methyl glucoside sesquistearate—an organic emulsifier obtained from a natural simple sugar.

Mineral oil—an organic emollient and lubricant.

Myristyl myristate—an emollient derived from an acid found in coconut oil and nutmeg butter and alcohol from naturally fatty acids.

Oleic acid—a lubricant usually derived from olive or coconut oil.

Olive oil—a natural oil obtained from olives.

Papain—a papaya enzyme.

Peanut oil—a vegetable oil obtained from peanuts.

Pectin—derived from citrus fruits and apple peel.

PEG lanolin—an emollient and emulsifier obtained from lanolin.

Petrolatum—petroleum jelly.

P.O.E. (20) methyl glucoside sesquistearate—an organic emulsifier from a simple natural sugar.

Polysorbate 60—a wax made from sorbitol and stearic acid (see below) and used as a stabilizer.

Potassium sorbate—obtained from sorbic acid found in the berries of mountain ash.

Propylene glycol—a glycerin-type alcohol often used to help bind water in many skin cosmetics.

Safflower oil-hybrid—a natural emollient obtained from a strain of specially cultivated plants.

Sesame oil—oil of pressed sesame seeds.

Sodium borate (Borax)—an inorganic natural mineral salt.

Sodium cetyl sulfate—a detergent and emulsifier obtained from coconut oil.

Sodium laureth sulfate—a detergent obtained from coconut oil.

Sodium lauryl sulfate—a detergent obtained from coconut oil.

Sodium PCA—a natural-occurring humectant found in the skin where it acts as the natural moisturizer.

Sorbic acid—a natural preservative derived from berries of mountain ash.

Sorbitan stearate—a combination of sorbitol and stearic acid.

Sorbitol—a moisturizing agent and humectant derived from fruits, berries, or algae.

Squalene—a moisturizer made from shark-liver oil.

Stearic acid—a white fatty acid found in solid animal fats and a few vegetable fats.

Titanium dioxide—natural inorganic mineral used as white pigment.

Tocopherol—a natural vitamin E.

Undecylenamide DEA—a natural preservative derived from castor oil.

Water—the universal solvent, and the major constituent of all living material.

Witch hazel—an astringent herbal extract rich in tannin.

107. Any Questions About Chapter V?

Over the past two years, I seem to have developed ridges

on my fingernails. Have you any idea what might have caused them, and are there any vitamins I can take to get rid of them?

Acute illness or fevers can cause ridges to form in the nails. This is usually because the stress of the disease depletes the body of needed nutrients— particularly vitamins A, B complex, folic acid, calcium, iron, and protein. I'd advise a supplement of vitamin B complex, 100 mg., 1–3 times daily; a high-potency multiple vitamin with chelated minerals with either breakfast or dinner; and vitamin A, 10,000 IU, daily, after any meal, 5 days a week.

Why is it supposed to be better for your hair to alternate shampoos every couple of weeks?

Probably because the cleansing and conditioning ingredients in most shampoos can—and do—build up, causing an overload that could deprive your hair of the bounce and sheen for which you bought the shampoo in the first place. Rinsing your hair with a solution of plain apple-cider vinegar and water can eliminate unwanted residue, and save you the expense (and bathroom shelf space) of numerous new shampoos. This is particularly important if you wash your hair consistently with hard water, which has more metal ions, and, when combined with soap, leaves a residue.

I've been told that seaweed is good for the skin. Looking at that yucky stuff that's washed ashore, I find it hard to believe. I'm always game for new natural beauty treatments, but this one seems hokey. Do you know anything about it?

I do, indeed. Seaweed is essentially highly concentrated sea water, with a large mineral content of magnesium, potassium, calcium, iodine, sodium, and particularly sulfur, which attracts moisture to the skin. It's often used as a dry skin treatment, since its amino acids and vitamins rectify skin deficiencies and aid in tissue development. I do not, though, recommend that you go to your local beach and gather up, as you call it, "that yucky stuff," for a home facial. Consult a professional, or find a reliable manufacturer of a seaweed-containing beauty product.

I hate using chemicals to bleach my hair, but I do like blonde streaks. I've tried lemon juice, but it just doesn't do enough. Are there any other natural hair lighteners?
    Chamomile oil! (You can find it at health food stores.) This is stronger than lemon juice, so try it on a few strands before combing through your hair all at once. For a milder, all-over lightening, use chamomile tea. Rinse your hair with it, then go outside and let the sun do the rest. (For reddish highlights, mix a bit of lemon juice with some brewed Red Zinger tea.)

TIME OUT

Fitness Subversives in Your Home

The following common household products, along with other indoor pollutants, have been found to be associated with a wide range of health problems—from mild nasal irritations and allergic reactions to toxic and carcinogenic effects.

PRODUCTS	WHAT THEY CONTAIN
Furniture polishes	Silicone, wax, and morpholine
Deodorant sprays	Hydrated aluminum chloride, talc, isopropylmyristate, and triclycerides
Hair sprays	Vinyl acetate copolymer resins, polyvinylpyrrolide resins, ethanol, and lanolin
Disinfectant sprays	Triisopropanolamine and morpholine
Window cleaners	Sodium nitrite, isopropyl alcohol, ethylene glycol, and ammonium hydroxide
Shaving foams	Stearic acid, thiethanolamine, menthol, and glycerine
Oven cleaners	Potassium hydroxide, hydroxyethyl cellulose, and polyoxyethylene fatty ethers
Air fresheners	Propylene glycol, morpholine, and ethanol

WHO Working Group,
Hidden Health Hazards in Our Environment.
April 1979

Think about it . . .

VI.

Feeling Great

108. Female Problems Farewell: Overcoming PMS

Though menstruation is a natural occurrence in a woman's life, PMS (premenstrual syndrome) is not. For two to ten days before the onset of menstruation, millions of women are afflicted with the symptoms of PMS, a wide range of physical discomforts and mood disorders that include bloating, blues, insomnia, severe abdominal pain, uncontrolled rages, crying spells, and even suicidal depression.

> Being nutritionally fit is a woman's best defense against PMS.

As with all illness, which PMS is, stress—and the inability of the body to combat it—is a key factor. Inadequate nutrition not only decreases resistance to stress but can even be the cause of it. Being nutritionally fit is a woman's best defense against PMS. But if you're already afflicted with the syndrome, knowing what and what not to eat is one of the most effective ways to fight back.

AVOID THESE FOODS AND BEVERAGES:

- Salt and salty foods (see section 62).
- Licorice (Licorice stimulates the production of aldosterone, which causes further retention of sodium and water.)
- Caffeine in all forms—coffee, chocolate, colas, and so on (Caffeine increases the craving for sugar, depletes B vitamins, washes out potassium and zinc, and increases hydrochloric acid [HCl] secretions, which can cause abdominal irritation.)
- Alcohol (Alcohol adversely affects blood sugar, depletes magnesium levels, and can interfere with proper liver function, aggravating PMS.)
- Astringent dark teas (Tannin binds important minerals and prevents absorption in the digestive tract.)
- Spinach, beet greens, and other oxalate-containing vegetables (Oxalates make minerals nonassimilable, difficult to be properly absorbed.)

INCREASE THESE FOODS AND BEVERAGES:

- Raw sunflower seeds, dates, figs, peaches. bananas, potatoes peanuts, and tomatoes (rich in potassium)
- Strawberries, watermelon (eat seeds), artichokes, asparagus, parsley, watercress (these are natural diuretics)
- Safflower, sunflower, sesame, or almond oil (2 tbsp. daily) or fish oil (2 tsp. daily) (Adequate amounts of essential fatty acids are required for the production of steroid hormones and prostaglandins, which have a marked effect on the uterus.)
- Figs, grapefruit, yellow corn, dark-green vegetables, apples (rich in magnesium, necessary for a healthy reproductive system, reduced during menstruation, and found in low levels among PMS sufferers)

SUGGESTED SUPPLEMENTS

- Vitamin B_6, 50–300 mg., daily (work up from 50 mg. gradually)
- MVP (See section 38.)
- Magnesium, 500 mg., and calcium, 250 mg., daily (Yes, with PMS the ratio should be twice as much magnesium as calcium because a magnesium deficiency causes many of the PMS symptoms.)
- Vitamin E (dry form) 200–400 IU, daily
- Pantothenic acid (vitamin B_5), 1,000 mg. (1 g.), daily (When taken with vitamin C, pantothenic acid helps to control allergic responses that can be more intense during the premenstrual time.)
- Evening primrose oil, 500 mg., 3 times daily (Helps alleviate pain as well as mood disorders brought on by PMS.)
- Dong quai, 2 caps, 3 times daily, ½ hour before or after meals (begin a week before menstruation) This herb is known as the female ginseng and can improve circulation, regulate liver function, and help remove excess water from the system.

RECOMMENDED EXERCISE

Sustained exercise (aerobic) is best. Brisk walking for thirty minutes twice daily (or swimming) is extremely effective in providing improved abdominal circulation and in minimizing PMS symptoms.

OTHER BENEFITS OF AEROBIC EXERCISE FOR PMS SUFFERERS:

- Helps prevent the retention of fluids

- Increases the level of beta endorphins in the brain (thus elevating mood)
- Aids in proper metabolization of needed nutrients
- Minimizes constipation and encourages regularity
- Helps reduce stress

109. Revitalizing Changes for the Change of Life

When a woman reaches menopause, somewhere around the age of fifty, her menstrual cycles cease, her production of the hormone estrogen declines, and a series of distressing physical and emotional symptoms usually occurs. Among these are hot flashes (sudden flushes or waves of heat and drenching sweat over the upper body), depression, vaginal dryness, urinary incontinence, increased risk of heart attack, and progressive bone deterioration.

Unfortunately, many doctors consider menopause a disease, instead of a natural process, and quickly prescribe estrogen (or related hormones) to treat change-of-life discomforts. But though estrogen replacement therapy (ERT), which employs such drugs as Tace (chlorotrianisene), Premarin (conjugated estrogens), Ogen (estropipate), and Estinyl (ethinyl estradiol) among others, is effective in treating moderate to severe vasomotor symptoms, such as hot flashes and the drying of vaginal mucous membranes, there is no evidence that it is effective in treating nervous symptoms or depression or in preventing heart attacks. And it has been found to be only "probably" effective in treating estrogen-deficiency-induced osteoporosis (bone deterioration), and then only when used with other therapeutic measures. On the other hand, *there IS evidence that these estrogens can increase the risk of endometrial cancer!* Additionally, women who've been on estrogen therapy often find that it only delays symptoms, such as hot flashes, which then seem to reappear when the drug is discontinued.

NOW, THE GOOD NEWS

- The hormonal imbalance that occurs at menopause is temporary, much like the changes that occur at puberty.
- No more than 10 to 20 percent of women going through menopause suffer extreme discomfort.
- Hot flashes usually last no more than two years, and, as a general rule, are *not* incapacitating.

NATURAL REVITALIZING REGIMEN

GINSENG: Helps alleviate hot flashes (often limiting them to eight weeks). Though containing estriol, a variant of estrogen, ginseng is an anticarcinogenic (anticancer) substance. As a supplement, I'd recommend 500 mg., taken on an empty stomach, A.M. and P.M. (Vitamin C has been said to diminish ginseng's effectiveness; but taking a time-release C supplement will make counteraction less likely.)

VITAMIN E (WITH SELENIUM): Helps alleviate menopausal symptoms by interacting with thyroid secretions and estrogen, moderating hormonal fluctuations. Both vitamin E and selenium are antioxidants, slowing down aging and tissue-hardening due to oxidation. They're also synergistic, which means that the action of the two combined produces an effect more potent than either would alone. I'd suggest starting with 200 IU and increasing to 400 IU (mixed tocopherols preferred), 1 to 3 times daily.

L-tryptophan: One of nature's pharmacy's best antidepressants and sedatives, and enormously helpful to women going through menopause. As a supplement, I'd recommend 3 tablets, (667 mg.), ½ hour before bedtime, taken with water or juice (no protein).

Calcium and magnesium: Aside from being effective natural tranquilizers, calcium and magnesium can help in the prevention and treatment of osteoporosis (the porous bone disease caused by demineralization due to lack of estrogen), backache, and muscle cramps that often cause insomnia during menopause. As a supplement, I'd suggest 1 chelated calcium (500 mg.) and magnesium (250 mg.) tablet, 3 times daily.

B-complex vitamins: These are your best insurance against the adverse emotional and physical effects of stress. (In fact, there is increasing evidence that an adequate B-complex vitamin intake throughout life helps prevent menopausal symptoms.) As a supplement, I'd suggest taking a stress B complex, 100 mg., 1–3 times daily.

Herb teas: For a soothing, mood-elevating drink, chamomile (and chamomile-based) tea is highly recommended. Teas containing passion flower (passiflora) are also helpful and work as effective sleeping aids. Valerian is another calming herb— and a potent one. If using the root to make tea, add only half a teaspoon to a cup of boiling water, then let it cool. Drink only one cup a day—and no more than a mouthful at a time.

Exercise: Brisk walking will tone up the circulatory system and can even prevent bone loss and strengthen the ligaments between bones. Swimming and bike-riding are also effective, as is jumping rope. (*CAUTION: Check with your doctor before beginning any sort of exercise* *regimen*.) I'd suggest fifteen minutes a day or a half-hour three times a week.

110. Sidestepping Osteoporosis

Osteoporosis (porous or brittle bones) is a degenerative condition characterized by the weakening of bones due to a slow but progressively accelerating loss of calcium, the essential mineral for strong bones. But this condition, which is reaching epidemic proportions in older women and is responsible for millions of fractures and thousands of deaths each year, *can be prevented*!

BONING UP ON THE FACTS

- Lowered estrogen levels lead to bone loss. (The earlier menopause occurs, the more likely you are to develop osteoporosis.)
- White women are more prone to osteoporosis than men and black or Hispanic females, who have greater bone density.
- Thin, postmenopausal, inactive women who smoke are at the highest risk for osteoporosis. (Bone loss after menopause occurs 50 percent faster among smokers.)
- Anorexic women, of any age, are probably candidates for osteoporosis.
- Excessive coffee drinking can interfere with calcium absorption and contribute to increased bone loss.
- A very high protein diet (95 mg. or more per day) can cause a loss of calcium and promote bone degeneration.
- Young women who exercise or diet excessively (to the extent that it causes a cessation of menstruation) become particularly vulnerable to osteoporosis.
- Vegetarians are less prone to osteoporosis than meat eaters.

- Efficient calcium absorption can be inhibited by tannic acid (in tea) as well as by oxalic acid (found in spinach, rhubarb, and beet greens, among other vegetables) and by phytic acid (found primarily in grains). Ironically, many of these foods are rich in calcium but aren't recommended as primary bone-building sources.
- Calcium absorption and availability can also be impeded by drugs such as aspirin, tetracyclines, furosemide diuretics (Lasix), anticonvulsant medications, aluminum-containing antacids, and the anticoagulant heparin, among others.
- Tooth loss from periodontal disease could be an early warning sign of osteoporosis.
- The current 800 mg. calcium recommended daily allowance (RDA) for women is 200–700 mg. below what bone experts deem sufficient for adequate calcium balance.

℞ FOR NATURAL PREVENTION

- Keep your calcium intake up! *At least* 1,000 mg. daily if premenopausal and 1,500 mg. daily if postmenopausal.
- Increase your intake of such foods as yogurt, sardines (bones included), salmon, carrot juice (see section 36 for other calcium-rich foods), and supplement with 3 chelated calcium and magnesium tablets, 3 times daily (A.M., P.M., and ½ hour before bedtime).
- Avoid excessive consumption of soft drinks, processed foods, and meat.
- To aid calcium absorption, a supplement of vitamin D, 800 IU, daily is advised, as well as 1,000 mg. of vitamin C.
- Exercise *regularly*! (Best bets are walking, bicycling, swimming, and rope-jumping.) Minimum exercise time

should be 20 minutes, 3 times a week. This can actually *strengthen* bones!

111. Snapping Back After Surgery

No matter what sort of surgery you've had, your body has gone through a trauma and stress has taken its nutritional toll on you.

To speed the healing process and get you back to feeling fit *fast*, the following supplements, taken in conjunction with a balanced diet and adequate rest, can work wonders:

- Vitamin E, 400 IU (dry form), 3 times daily
- Vitamin C complex, 1,000 mg. with bioflavonoids, hesperidin, and rutin, A.M. and P.M.
- Vitamin B complex, 50–100 mg., 1–3 times daily
- High-potency multiple vitamin with chelated minerals, A.M. and P.M.
- High-potency multiple chelated mineral tablet, A.M. and P.M.
- Vitamin A, 10,000–25,000 IU, 3 times daily for 5 days (stop for 2 days to prevent buildup)
- Chelated zinc, 15–50 mg., daily

112. Strategies for Livelier Living with Arthritis

There are many forms and causes of arthritis, which is basically an inflammation of a joint or joints. It can strike persons of any age, be caused by injury as well as by a complication of another disease (e.g., rubella), exist as a symptom accompanying a systemic infection, and even occur as a side effect of certain medications—particularly contraceptives, anticonvulsants, and major tranquilizers.

> Arthritis can strike at any age...and even occur as a side effect of certain medications!

Osteoarthritis and rheumatoid arthritis are only two of approximately one hundred conditions known as rheumatic diseases, which encompass tendinitis, hepatitis, gout, syphilis, diabetes mellitus, and more.

But diet and exercise can help! Though conclusive evidence is not yet in, there have been enough established correlations between arthritic diseases and nutrition to convince me and thousands of former arthritis sufferers that knowing what and what not to eat (as well as how and when to exercise) can mean the difference between being housebound and fitness bound.

ARTHRITIS DEFENSE

DIET:
- Avoid coffee, tea, soft drinks, sugar, alcohol, and all refined carbohydrates.
- Increase your intake of vegetables (see section 144 for how to get the most vitamins from them).
- Eat more raw vegetables.
- Exclude foods in the nightshade family of vegetables, such as potatoes, tomatoes, and eggplant, among others.
- Increase your intake of vitamin-C-rich foods (see section 36). Arthritis is essentially a collagen disease, and vitamin C is necessary for the formation of collagen.

SUPPLEMENTS:
- High-potency multiple vitamin with chelated minerals (time release preferred), A.M. and P.M.
- High-potency chelated multiple mineral, A.M. and P.M.
- Vitamin C, 1,000 mg., 1–3 times daily (if you take aspirin, you're losing a *lot* of vitamin C)

- Vitamin B complex, 100 mg., 1–3 times daily
- Vitamin B$_{12}$, 100–200 mcg., daily
- Niacin, 50–500 mg., daily
- Yucca tabs, or alfalfa tabs, 1–3, 3 times daily
- Pantothenic acid, 100 mg., 3 times daily
- Vitamin A, 10,000 IU, 3 times daily for 5 days (stop for 2)
- Vitamin D, 400 IU, 3 times daily for 5 days (stop for 2), or cod-liver oil, 1–2 tbsp., 3 times daily (if capsules, 3 caps, 3 times daily) Again, take for 5 days and stop for 2.

EXERCISE:

It's true that inflammation is reduced by rest, but too much rest can cause tendons to weaken and bones to soften, while exercise can relieve pain, strengthen endurance, and prevent arthritic conditions from worsening.

Find a doctor qualified to design a personalized exercise program that's suited to your individual needs and abilities. Your local arthritis foundation should be able to recommend one.

After consulting with a physician, find ways to incorporate exercise into your daily routine.

Avoid exercise that puts a burden on weight-bearing joints (tennis, jogging, and so on), and think more about activities such as swimming or yoga.

Keep your weight down to avoid unnecessary stress on joints.

Keep up a regular sex life. Sex can act as a pain reliever, according to Dr. Jessie E. Potter, director of the National Institute for Human Relationships, through adrenal stimulation. Any kind of sexual arousal—self-stimulation, petting, oral sex—leads to cortisone release and can give patients from four to six hours of relief from arthritis pain.

113. Revving-up Your Immune System— Why It's Necessary

As you get older, your immune system—a stalwart, ever-ready army of white blood cells (called T-cells because they're under the command of the thymus gland), which has been instructed where and when to attack and what antibodies their cofighters (called B-cells because they're made in the bone marrow) should produce—begins to break down due to the decreasing power and size of the thymus gland. This causes not only an ineffectual defense system but often an unwittingly mutinous one.

> As you get older, your immune system can turn against you.

With the breakdown of command, dangerous confusion occurs, causing T-cells to mistake friends for enemies. And when this happens, instead of fighting off invaders, they attack you! The result can be any of numerous autoimmune disorders (AIDS among them), as well as such diseases as multiple sclerosis, myesthenia gravis, and arthritis. Because recent research has shown that this breakdown is most likely due to a reduced rate of growth hormone, which is produced by the pituitary gland and necessary to the function of the thymus gland and therefore the immune system, dietary reinforcements and supplements have been deemed indispensable in reversing this degenerative syndrome.

THE RIGHT FUEL

Vitamin A, 10,000–25,000 IU, daily, 5 days a week (stop for 2)
Stimulates immune system; helps prevent shrinkage of thymus gland.

Vitamin C, 1,000 mg., 1–3 times daily
> Effective immune-system stimulant; aids in preventing numerous viral, bacterial, and cancer infections by increasing activity of certain white cells.

Vitamin E (dry form), 200–400 IU, 1–3 times daily
> Effective immune-system stimulant; aids in combatting viruses, bacteria, and cancer cells.

Arginine, 2,000 mg., daily (take with water, no protein, and on an empty stomach)
> Aids immune system; necessary for release of growth hormone; helps block formation of tumors.

Ornithine, 2,000 mg., daily (with water, no protein, and on an empty stomach)
> Increases levels of arginine in the body, further aids immune system and stimulates release of growth hormone; helps insulin work as an anabolic (muscle-building hormone).

Cysteine, 1 gram daily with vitamin C 3 grams (3 times as much vitamin C as cysteine)
> An anti-aging amino acid that helps protect body from destructive free radicals.

Selenium, 50–100 mcg., daily
> Retards aging; works synergistically with vitamin E (making vitamin E a more effective immune-system stimulant).

Zinc, chelated, 15–50 mg., 1–3 times daily
> Helps prevent shrinkage of thymus gland; works best with vitamin A, calcium, and phosphorus; oversees the efficient flow of body processes, the maintenance of enzyme systems and cells.

Propolis, 500 mg., 1–3 times daily
> Stimulates the thymus gland, enhancing the body's immune system.

Papain
> An enzyme found in papaya that stimulates the production of early-forming immune system cells.

Interleukin 2

Stimulates production of T-cells and "immune interferon," a group of antiviral proteins; may be a factor in cancer prevention. (Not available in U.S.A. at this writing.)

EXERCISE!

Regular exercise increases the number of your white blood cells (infection fighters). In fact, because vigorous exercise raises body temperature, it can work much like a fever (which many doctors now feel is an important defense against infection because fevers can inhibit the growth of microorganisms).

114. Don't Let Diabetes Get You Down

Diabetes occurs when the body is unable to fully metabolize sugars and starches, either because the pancreas doesn't produce enough insulin for processing, or the insulin produced is less than effective.

In mild cases, diet alone can control the condition. In severe cases, replacement insulin is necessary. In all cases, the care of a physician is essential— but that doesn't mean you have to give up on your get-up-and-go!

ENERGIZE YOUR EATING

- Keep your diet low in fats and high in complex carbohydrates, especially those that are rich in fiber, such as whole grains and dried beans.
- Avoid all foods containing refined sugars.
- Have 4–6 small meals daily instead of 2–3 large ones.
- Eat more fish. It's high in protein and low in fat.

- Increase raw fruits and vegetables in your diet.
- Add brewer's yeast to meals when you can— especially if you're a senior citizen. (Impaired glucose tolerance is a definite factor in maturity-onset diabetes, and brewer's yeast is a prime source of GTF, the glucose tolerance factor which can potentiate insulin.)
- Make sure your meals contain plenty of vitamin E- and C-rich foods (see section 36). These will help counteract the poor circulation and impeded blood vessels that diabetics are prone to.
- Drink a cup of freshly made blueberry tea 2–3 times daily (steep leaves in hot water for half an hour). It's one of the best herbal remedies for lowering blood sugar.

SUGGESTED SUPPLEMENTS

- MVP (see section 38)
- GTF chromium, 200 mcg., 3 times daily (see Caution, section 64)
- Potassium, 99 mg., 3 times daily
- Chelated zinc, 50 mg., 1–3 times daily
- Water, 6–8 glasses daily
  AND DON'T FORGET EXERCISE!

115. Taking Action Against Allergies

Few things can undermine fitness faster than allergies, which stem from innumerable causes and cause reactions ranging from headaches, colds, and rashes to asthmatic attacks and even anaphylactic shock.

An allergy is a natural immunity that's gone amock.

Basically, an allergy is a natural immunity that's gone amock. A seemingly harmless substance, for instance, can—in some people—cause the immune system to create excessive antibodies when none are needed, resulting in a variety of debilitating and discomforting symptoms.

YOUR BEST DEFENSE

- MVP (see section 38) A.M. and P.M.
- Vitamin B complex, 100 mg., 3 times daily
- Pantothenic acid, 1,000 mg., A.M. and P.M.

Unless you're absolutely sure of the offending allergen, avoid highly allergenic foods, such as shellfish, chocolate, and eggs, as well as any containing additives, preservatives, food colorings, or MSG.

Anyone with a sulfite allergy (see section 120) must be extremely careful in selecting foods; adverse reactions can be lethal.

116. Fitness for Asthmatics

Asthma, a chronic allergic condition (attributed to numerous physiological, emotional, and genetic causes), affects the bronchial tubes, squeezing the air passage and causing labored breathing and a feeling of suffocation.

Because of this, asthmatics were formerly severely restricted in their activities. But recent research has shown that this was not merely an overreactive precaution but a detrimental one as well, depriving asthma sufferers of substantial exercise benefits.

Though strenuous sports such as tennis, soccer, football, basketball, and the like are still contraindicated, swimming and calisthenics (particularly those that enhance chest muscles and diaphragm) are now viewed, in most cases, as quite beneficial. (ALWAYS CHECK WITH YOUR DOCTOR BEFORE STARTING ANY EXERCISE.)

Additionally, the following supplements have been found to provide remarkable natural relief. (*See cautions for this regimen below.*)

- MVP (see section 38) A.M. and P.M.
- Extra vitamin C, 1,000 mg., 1–3 times daily
- Evening primrose oil (EPO), 2-500 mg. capsules, 3 times daily for 3 to 4 months; then 1 capsule 3 times daily. (If taking steroids, you won't benefit from EPO, because steroids interfere with EPO's action.)
- Glandulars (adrenal gland concentrates), 1–3 times daily
- Vitamin A (water soluble), 10,000–25,000 IU, daily (5 days a week)
- Vitamin B_2 (riboflavin), 100 mg., 3–4 times daily
- Vitamin B_5 (pantothenic acid), 1,000–2,000 mg., daily
- Vitamin B_6 (pyridoxine), 100 mg., 1–3 times daily
- Vitamin E (dry form), 400–1,200 IU daily

CAUTIONS FOR ASTHMA SUPPLEMENTS:

- Vitamin C that's buffered with calcium ascorbate can interfere with the action of tetracyclines. A sodium ascorbate form of vitamin C can be used with tetracyclines, but *not* if you're on a sodium-restricted diet or taking steroids.
- Glandulars, which shouldn't be taken at night because they could cause insomnia, should not be taken by anyone who's allergic to beef or pork.

117. Battling Yeast Infections—And Winning!

Yeast infections (candida albicans) are prevalent, debilitating, and conquerable.

When the candida or yeast germ gets out of control in the body, it produces a toxin that not only affects the nervous system (causing headaches, fatigue, depression, hyperactivity, and memory loss, among others) but also the reproductive organs, leading to abdominal pain, persistent vaginitis, bladder problems, loss of sexual interest, and more.

CAUSES

- Antibiotics
- Nutritional deficiencies
- Birth control pills or cortisone
- Diabetes mellitus
- Improper hygiene
- Anxiety or physical stress
- Chronic constipation or diarrhea
- Food or chemical allergies

CURES

- Avoid substances that yeast can thrive on, such as sugar and refined carbohydrates.
- Eliminate all yeast-containing foods and any that may have mold (for at least several weeks or until the infection is gone). These include cheese, raised breads, sour cream, buttermilk, beer, wine, cider, mushrooms, soy sauce, tofu, vinegar, dried fruits, melons, frozen or canned juices.
- The drug usually prescribed is Nystatin, but there are many natural and extremely effective dietary combatants. Among them are garlic, broccoli, cabbage, onions, plain yogurt, turnips and other vegetables.

SUPPLEMENTS

- High-potency multiple vitamin, A.M. and P.M.
- High-potency chelated multiple minerals (with at least 1,000 mg. calcium and 500 mg. magnesium, as well as adequate amounts of iron, zinc, and selenium)
- High potency acidophilus capsule or 1 tbsp. of acidophilus liquid (flavored) 1–3 times daily
- Vitamin C, 1,000 mg. (time release), A.M. and P.M.
- Vitamin E (dry form), 200–400 IU, daily
- Propolis, 500 mg., 3 times daily
- Free-form amino acids (balanced formula) daily

118. Conditioning Your Heart

Anyone with a heart condition—or who suspects one— should be under a doctor's care. But the following prevention tactics could help you from ever needing it.

- Decrease your consumption of sugar, salt, saturated fats, hydrogenated oils, and cholesterol
- Watch your weight
- Stop smoking
- Practice relaxation techniques such as meditation and biofeedback to reduce stress
- Eat more garlic, fresh fruit, and fish
- Increase your intake of soy protein (use in place of animal protein whenever possible)
- Get enough calcium and magnesium in your diet (supplements of 1,000 mg. calcium and 500 mg. magnesium daily are recommended)
- Laugh more (it really is the best medicine)
- EXERCISE REGULARLY

SUPPLEMENT SUGGESTIONS

- MVP (see section 38)
- Vitamin B complex, 100 mg. (time release), A.M. and P.M.

- Extra niacin, 100 mg., 1–3 times daily (Caution: Flushing, itching, and tingling skin sensations can occur in sensitive individuals.)
- Vitamin E (dry form), 400 IU, daily
- 3 lecithin capsules (1,200 mg.), or 3 tbsp. granules, 3 times daily

CAUTION: If you are on *any* heart medication, check with your doctor before starting a supplement regimen. Also, be aware that vitamin E can increase the imbalance between the two sides of the heart for some people with rheumatic hearts.

119. Some Simple Shape-ups for Special Problems That Can Get You Down

COLDS

- MVP (see section 38)
- Vitamin C complex, 1,000 mg., 3 times daily
- Vitamin A, 25,000 IU, 1–3 times daily for 5 days, then stop for 2
- Vitamin E (dry form), 200–400 IU, daily
- Water, 6–8 glasses daily
- 3 acidophilus capsules, 3 times daily, or ½ tbsp. liquid, 3 times daily
- Zinc lozenges, 15 mg., dissolve in mouth 3 times daily

COLITIS

- MVP (see section 38)
- Potassium, 99 mg. (elemental), 1–3 times daily
- Raw cabbage juice (vitamin U), 1 glass, 3 times daily

- Water, 6–8 glasses daily
- Aloe vera (for internal use), 1 tbsp., 3 times daily, or 1–3 capsules, 3 times daily
- 3–6 acidophilus caps, 3 times daily, or 2 tbsp. liquid, 3 times daily
- 1 tbsp. bran flakes, 3 times daily, or 3–6 bran tablets, 3 times daily

HAY FEVER

- Stress B complex, 100 mg., twice daily
- Pantothenic acid, 1,000 mg., 3 times daily
- Vitamin C, 1,000 mg., 3 times daily

HIGH BLOOD PRESSURE (HYPERTENSION)

- Decrease sodium and increase potassium in your diet.
- Reduce if you're overweight.
- Talk slower (fast talkers often don't breathe properly and this can elevate blood pressure)
- Decrease intake of sugar.
- Stop smoking and eliminate caffeine.
- Eat more onions and garlic.
- Avoid stress or anxiety-provoking situations.
- Exercise regularly (see "walking" section 19)
- Check with your doctor or a nutritionally oriented physician (see section 145) regularly.
- Lecithin granules, 3 tbsp. daily, or 3 caps, 3 times daily
- MVP (see section 38)
- Calcium, 1,000–1,500 mg., daily
- Vitamin E, 100 IU, daily, and work up to higher strengths (check with doctor)
- Garlic capsules (deodorized), 1–3 daily

- Potassium supplements may be necessary if you are taking an antihypertensive medication, but check with your doctor to be sure that it's not contraindicated for your particular drug.

HYPOGLYCEMIA

- Eat smaller, more frequent meals, high in protein and complex carbohydrates
- Vitamin A and D capsules, (10,000 and 400 IU), 1–3 times daily for 5 days, then stop for 2
- Vitamin C, 500 mg., with or after each meal
- Vitamin E, 100–200 IU, 3 times daily
- B complex, 50 mg., 3 times daily
- Vitamin F, 1 cap, 3 times daily
- Multiple mineral tab, A.M. and P.M.
- Pantothenic acid, 500 mg., twice daily
- 2 lecithin capsules (19 grains = 1,200 mg.), 3 times daily
- 1 kelp tab, 3 times daily
- 3 acidophilus capsules, or 1–2 tbsp. liquid, 3 times daily
- GTF chromium, 200 mcg., 3 times daily
- Digestive enzymes, if necessary

JET LAG

- Stress B complex (time release), A.M. and P.M. (start while still on the plane)
- MVP (see section 38) with food (twice during flights of 5 or more hours)
- Vitamin E (dry form), 400 IU, twice daily
- Extra vitamin C, if necessary

MIGRAINES

- Practice relaxation techniques such as biofeedback and meditation.
- Try to avoid taking oral contraceptives or estrogen supplements.
- Keep away from foods with additives, caffeine, and alcoholic beverages.
- Increase your intake of niacin-rich foods (see section 36). Niacin has been found to help prevent and ease the severity of migraine headaches.
- Supplement your diet with Vitamin B complex (time release), twice daily; calcium and magnesium (1,000 mg. calcium to 500 mg. magnesium), A.M. and P.M.
- Drink a cup of peppermint or sage tea, then lie down in a darkened room for 20 minutes.
- Exercise for relief by letting your head fall forward and *slowly* rotate it in a wide circle, 3 times clockwise and then 3 times counterclockwise. Rest, and then gently massage neck and back of head.
- Fever Few capsules 3 times daily. New research about an old herb showed its usefulness in migraines.

SHINGLES

- Vitamin A, 10,000–25,000 IU, daily for 5 days, then stop for 2
- Vitamin B complex, 100 mg. (time release), A.M. and P.M.
- Vitamin C complex, 1,000–2,000 mg., A.M. and P.M.
- Vitamin D, 1,000 IU, daily for 5 days, then stop for 2

120. Any Questions About Chapter VI?

Is it true that diabetic women are more prone to vaginal yeast infections?

Yes. It's because they have higher concentrations of sugar in their vaginal secretions.

My sister's doctor told her that her asthma attacks were caused by a "sulfite" sensitivity. Could you tell me what this is, and if it's dangerous? Also, I'd like to know why she was advised to keep away from, of all things, restaurant salad bars?

A sulfite sensitivity is not only dangerous, it can be deadly! It is an allergy to sulfites (sulfur dioxide, potassium or sodium bisulfite, potassium or sodium metabisulfite, and sodium sulfite), chemical preservatives widely used in beer, wine, restaurant and food-processing industries. Restaurants almost always use sulfiting agents to retard the discoloration of vegetables and sliced fruits, allowing them to keep the salad bar selections fresh-looking and appealing for hours—even days!

Asthmatics are at highest risk of life-threatening reactions, but millions of other sulfite-sensitive people are subject to hives, shortness of breath, fainting, and even death from these additives.

Anyone who suspects a sulfite sensitivity should read package labels carefully to be sure the product contains none of the above-named additives, and should avoid the following:

- Restaurant fresh fruit and vegetables cut up for buffets or salad bars
- Fresh shrimp and other shellfish (sulfites are often used to prevent unappetizing but harmless discolorations on shrimp)
- Most wines, and possibly some brands of beer (unfortunately, alcohol-labeling is not under the FDA's jurisdiction)
- Wine vinegar

- Restaurant-sliced potatoes, french fries, avocado, or cut-apple dishes
- Frozen pizza
- Dough and starch products (including Uncle Ben's Long Grain and Wild Rice)
- Dried fruits and vegetables.

Vitamin B_{12} has been found to diminish and even prevent asthmatic reactions to sulfites. I'd recommend that your sister take 2,000 mcg. sublingually daily. She should, of course, first check with her doctor—or a nutritionally oriented physician (see section 145).

TIME OUT

Growing Old

We do not grow old because our immune system fails. However, we deteriorate more rapidly the more our immune system becomes deranged as a result of ill health, nutritional imbalances, or both.

Hans Weber, Ph.D.
Healthline, February 1984

Think about it...

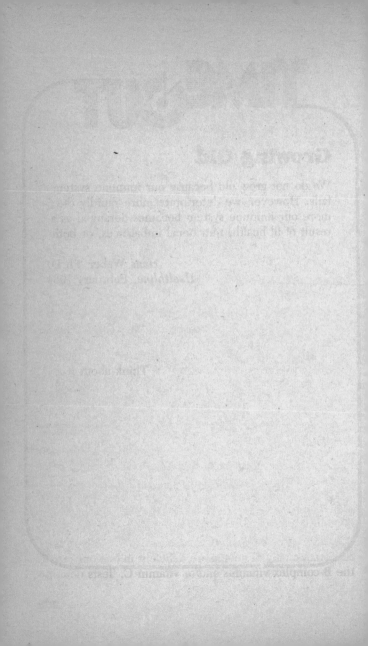

VII.

Emotion Energizing

121. What You Eat Can Pick You Up or Bring You Down

Biochemical causes for mental disturbances, once regarded by doctors as a farfetched theory, have now become accepted in myriad cases as virtual fact.

> The majority of mentally and emotionally ill people are deficient in one or more of the B-complex vitamins and/or vitamin C.

Numerous experiments have proved that many symptoms of mental illness can be switched off and on by altering vitamin levels in the body.

A study made by Dr. R. Shulman, reported in the *British Journal of Psychiatry*, found that forty-eight out of fifty-nine psychiatric patients had folic acid deficiencies. Other research has shown that the majority of mentally and emotionally ill people are deficient in one or more of the B-complex vitamins and/or vitamin C. Tests done by

Dr. Linus Pauling at California's Stanford University indicated that the mentally ill needed one thousand times the RDA of vitamin C than the rest of us require. In fact, even normal, happy people can become depressed when made deficient in niacin or folic acid.

122. Foods To Elevate Moods

SOME NUTRITIOUS UPPERS FROM NATURE'S PANTRY Whole wheat products, brewer's yeast, liver, kidney, wheat germ, fish, eggs, peanuts, the white meat of poultry, avocados, dates, figs, prunes, rice husks, oatmeal, bran, milk, green leafy vegetables, cantaloupe, cabbage, blackstrap molasses, lean meat, cheese, citrus fruits, berries, tomatoes, cauliflower, broccoli, brussels sprouts, ground mustard, potatoes, sweet potatoes, heart, soybeans, sardines, salmon, walnuts, sunflower seeds, dried beans, dairy products, yellow corn, almonds, nuts, apples, lemons, grapefruit, peas, beets, whole-grain cereals, bananas, turkey, cottage cheese, lima beans, and pumpkin and sesame seeds.

CAUTION: If you are allergic to gluten, avoid all products containing wheat, oats, rye, barley, or vegetables such as beans, cabbage, turnips, dried peas, and cucumbers, otherwise emotion-energizing results can be reversed. The same holds true if you are allergic to dairy or citrus products.

123. Nutrients That Fight Depression, Anxiety, and Stress

Vitamin B₁ Above-average amounts have been found
(thiamine) to tranquilize anxious individuals and
            alleviate depression.

Vitamin B$_6$ (pyridoxine)	Necessary for the function of the adrenal cortex and therefore proper production of natural antidepressants such as dopamine and norepinephrine.
Pantothenic acid	A natural tension-reliever when sufficient in diet.
Vitamin C (ascorbic acid)	Essential for combating stress.
Vitamin B$_{12}$ (cobalamin)	Helps relieve irritability, improve concentration, increase energy, and maintain a healthy nervous system.
Vitamin E (alpha-tocopherol)	Aids brain cells in getting needed oxygen.
Folic acid (colacin)	Essential for growth and reproduction of all body cells. A deficiency has been found to be a contributing factor in mental illness.
Zinc	Promotes mental alertness and aids in proper brain function.
Magnesium	Necessary for nerve-functioning, and known as the antistress mineral.
Niacin	A B-complex vitamin vital to the proper function of the nervous system.
Calcium	Alleviates tension, irritability, and promotes relaxation.
Tyrosine	An amino acid that releases a substance called catecholamine which, in turn, increases the rate at which brain neurons produce the antidepressants dopamine and norepinephrine.

| Tryptophan | An amino acid that works in conjunction with vitamin B_6, niacin, and magnesium to synthesize the vital brain chemical serotonin, a natural tranquilizer. |
| Phenylala-nine | An essential amino acid that's necessary for the the brain's release of the antidepressants dopamine and norepinephrine. |

124. L-PA (L-Phenylalanine)—The Greatest Natural Mood Elevator Yet!

L-PA which is the L (natural) form of the amino acid phenylalanine, already acknowledged as an effective analgesic for chronic pain conditions, in its D (synthetic) LPA form, has now been found to be 89 to 100 percent effective in the treatment of depression.

It increases the production of PEA (phenylethylamine), a natural brain stimulant that resembles amphetamine; elevates levels of endorphins (morphinelike hormones that have been alleged to account for the euphoria experienced by aerobic enthusiasts), and increases the production of norepinephrine, the mood-elevating brain chemical whose deficiency has been linked to severe depression.

SUPPLEMENT GUIDE

L-PA tabs (250-500 mg.), 3 daily, 1 hour before each meal. (When depression eases up, decrease to 1 tablet daily and then discontinue therapy.) If there is no improvement in 4–6 weeks, consult a nutritionally oriented physician (see section 145) and discontinue therapy.

CAUTION: Pregnant women or anyone who has PKU (phenylketonuria) should not use L-PA. Also, it should not be used in conjunction with any antidepressant medication that you are taking, *unless specifically cleared by your doctor.*

125. Bad Mood Bearers: Foods, Drugs, and Medications That Can Sink Your Spirits

FOODS	MOOD-REGULATING NUTRIENTS STOLEN
Refined sugars and carbohydrates	B-complex vitamins
Cakes, cookies, potato chips, pretzels, candy bars, chewing gum, sugared cereals, junk foods, etc.	B-complex vitamins
Chocolate, cocoa, all caffeine-containing beverages—colas, coffee, tea	B-complex vitamins, zinc; calcium assimilation inhibited
Processed foods and luncheon meats (bologna, hot dogs, ham, etc.) and any with artificial colorings or additives	B-complex vitamins

DRUGS AND MEDICINES

Alcohol (including alcohol-containing cough syrups, elixirs, and OTC medications such as Nyquil)	Vitamins B_1, B_2, choline, niacin, folic acid, and magnesium

DRUGS AND MEDICINES	MOOD-REGULATING NUTRIENTS STOLEN
Ammonium chloride (e.g., Ambenyl Expectorant, Triaminicol Decongestant Cough Syrup, P-V Tussin Syrup)	Vitamin C
Antacids (e.g., Maalox, Mylanta, Gelusil, Tums, Rolaids)	B-complex vitamins
Antihistamines	Vitamin C
Aspirin (and any APC drugs)	B-complex vitamins, vitamin C, calcium
Barbiturates (e.g., Phenobarbital, Seconal, Nembutal)	Vitamin C, folic acid
Caffeine (in all APC drugs)	B-complex vitamins, zinc; calcium assimilation inhibited
Chloramphenicol (Chloromycetin)	Niacin
Diuretics (e.g., Diuril, Lasix, Ser-Ap-Es)	B-complex vitamins, zinc, magnesium
Fluorides	Vitamin C
Glutethimide (Doriden)	Folic acid
Indomethacin (Indocin)	Vitamins B_1 and C
Isoniazid (INH, Nydrazid)	Vitamin B_6
Laxatives, lubricant	Calcium
Meprednisone (Betapar)	Vitamins B_6, C, zinc

DRUGS AND MEDICINES	MOOD-REGULATING NUTRIENTS STOLEN
Methotrexate (Mexate)	Folic acid
Nitrofurantoin (e.g., Furadantin, Macrodantin)	Folic acid
Oral contraceptives	Folic acid, vitamins B_6 and C
Penicillamine (Cuprimine)	Vitamin B_6
Penicillin (all forms)	Vitamin B_6, niacin
Phenylbutazone (e.g., Azolid, Butazolidin)	Folic acid
Phenytoin (Dilantin)	Folic acid
Prednisone (e.g., Meticorten, Orasone)	Vitamins B_6, C, zinc
Pyrimethamine (Daraprim)	Folic acid
Sulfonamides, systemic (e.g., Bactrim, Gantrisin, Septra)	Folic acid
Sulfonamides and topical steroids (e.g., Aerosporin, Cortisporin, Polysporin)	Folic acid
Tetracyclines (e.g., ACH-Romycin-V, Sumycin, Tetracyn)	Calcium, magnesium
Tobacco (nicotine)	Vitamins B_1, C, folic acid, calcium
Triamterene (Dyrenium)	Folic acid

126. Un-stressing for Success

Studies of the effects of stress, whether physical (hunger, fatigue, pain) or emotional (grief, anxiety, anger), have shown that it leads to the release of catecholamines (such as epinephrine and norepinephrine), "fight or flight" hormones, which in turn effect other bodily changes, straining the cardiovascular system and weakening our resistance to disease.

ILLNESSES THAT HAVE BEEN LINKED TO STRESS

Heart disease	Cancer
Hypertension	Diabetes
Migraines	Allergies
Backaches	Rheumatoid arthritis
Herpes recurrence	Cirrhosis
Suicidal depression	Colds
Mononucleosis	Influenza
Skin breakouts	(and more)

Occasional stress is normal in everyone's life, but chronic or cumulative stress can dangerously undermine the function of your immune system.

HOW TO UN-STRESS

- Think positively—laughter really is great medicine.
- Practice relaxation techniques—meditation, biofeedback.
- Get enough exercise. (A relaxed muscle can't be tense, and pleasurable exercise produces relaxed muscles.)
- Get enough rest.
- Avoid caffeine.
- Drink lots of liquids. (Cutting down on food intake

during extremely stressful periods allows your digestive organs to rest, freeing that energy to help your body's healing systems.)

- Try a glass of warm milk before bedtime; it's a fine source of typtophan (an essential amino acid that aids in reducing anxiety and tension). For other good sources of tryptophan, see section 36.
- Increase foods rich in B vitamins, niacin, PABA, and magnesium in your daily diet. (See section 36.)
- Stress speeds up potassium loss, so be sure to eat enough potassium-rich foods; bananas, potatoes, and citrus fruits are terrific sources.
- A glass of celery juice daily can be a refreshing un-stresser.
- A soothing cup of herb tea made of equal parts hops, lavender flowers, balm leaves, and primrose, taken by mouthfuls as needed, has a natural calming effect.

SUPPLEMENTS SUGGESTED

- Stress B complex with vitamin C, 1–3 times daily
- Chelated calcium and magnesium, 3 tabs, 3 times daily
- L-tryptophan, 500–667 mg., 1–3 times daily (with water, no protein)
- Propolis, 500 mg.; take 15 to 20 minutes before each meal (preferably on an empty stomach), 1–3 times daily.

127. Don't Overwind Your Body Clock
Inside all of us is what has been described as a "master timekeeper"—a multifunction body clock that regulates everything from our metabolism to our moods.

According to Dr. Charles F. Stroebel, director of the Institute for Advanced Studies in Behavioral Medicine, Hartford, Connecticut, "Recognition of the role of body time in regulating health may eventually prevent 90 percent of all illnesses."

Some functions of our body clocks—the sleep and wake ones in particular—are easily affected by stress or sickness, darkness and light, even our own work, play, and rest schedules.

> A couple of late nights in a row can throw your body clock off—reducing your alertness, energy, and disease resistance for days... sometimes weeks!

Studies done by Dr. Charles P. Pollak, head of the Sleep-Wake Disorders Center at the Westchester Division of the New York Hospital-Cornell Medical Center, have shown that something as simple as exercising right before bedtime can throw your body clock out of sync, causing insomnia, depriving the body of the time when it normally recharges its energy supply. In fact, a couple of late nights on the town in a row can throw your body clock off to the point of reducing your alertness, energy, and resistance to disease for days (and in some cases weeks). You can't just rewind your body clock, it needs time to readjust to changes in schedule. (For supplements that can help, see section 119 on jet lag.)

If you must do something that interferes with your regular sleep-wake routine, Dr. Stroebel suggests following your usual schedule for several days beforehand, then making your changes (either going to bed earlier or later) gradually.

Biorhythms are still rhythms—and interrupting them takes its toll emotionally and physically. Your best nutritional defense is to keep your diet high in stress-reducing foods (those rich in all the B vitamins, vitamin C, calcium, magnesium, zinc, tyrosine, tryptophan, and phenylalanine). And a daily MVP supplement (see section 38) is essential.

128. Alcohol: Why "Bottoms Up!" Can Be a Real Downer

Hoisting a glass of alcohol will not, contrary to popular belief (and forgive the pun) lift your spirits. Though you might think, after that first drink, that you feel great, alcohol only creates the illusion of stimulation. It is *not* a stimulant, it is a central-nervous-system *depressant!*

Because alcohol requires no digestion, it passes directly into the bloodstream, increases circulation to the nerve centers of the brain, and produces intoxication, dulling inhibitions and providing a temporary release from anxiety. After that, it's downhill all the way.

THINK BEFORE YOU DRINK

- Alcohol depletes the body of B vitamins (especially folic acid) as well as substantial amounts of calcium, magnesium, zinc, and other trace minerals, all of which are essential emotion energizers.
- It impairs coordination and reduces contractile strength of muscles.
- It interferes with nutrient absorption and destroys enzymes necessary for good health and fitness.
- It impedes formation and storage of glycogen in the liver; in other words, cuts down your fitness fuel.
- It increases your risk of infection and worsens allergic reactions to foods.
- Chronic use results in loss of brain cells, causing memory lapses, impaired learning ability, motor disturbances, and general disorientation.

- Pregnant women who drink endanger their unborn children with Fetal Alcohol Syndrome, which can cause, aside from low birth weight, brain damage and physical malformation.
- Anyone who has acquired a tolerance to alcohol might need larger doses of sedatives or tranquilizers to attain the desired effect, increasing the possibility of an unwitting overdose.
- Alcohol can interact adversely with more than one hundred medications—with effects ranging from simple nausea to sudden death. Unless you've asked and been told by your physician that you can have a drink with another drug—DON'T!

129. Decreasing Your Desire for Alcohol with Nutrients

Niacin (vitamin B_3) has been found to be one of the most therapeutic agents in the treatment of alcoholism, especially when taken in conjunction with all the other B vitamins—particularly vitamins B_1, B_6, B_{12}, choline, and inositol. (See section 36 for foods containing these nutrients.)

Eating right can mean drinking less.

Research at the University of Texas by Professor Roger Williams has shown that if alcoholic mice are fed nutritious, vitamin-enriched diets, they quickly lose interest in alcohol. And the same seems to hold true with people. In other words, eating right can mean drinking less.

Dr. H. L. Newbold of New York recommends building up to five glutamine capsules (200 mg.)—not glutamic acid—three times a day to control drinking, but advises doing this only while under treatment with a nutritionally oriented physician (see section 145).

Serotonin, a natural tranquilizing substance in the brain, has been shown to be reduced in alcoholism. For this reason, supplements of L-tryptophan, an essential amino acid that's used by the brain (along with vitamin B₆, niacin, and magnesium) to produce serotonin, can help heavy drinkers break the habit by reducing their alcohol-related body chemistry disorders. Suggested L-tryptophan dose is 500 mg.–3 g. at bedtime (with water or juice, no protein).

130. Why Those Coffee Breaks Can Break You

Yes, that first cup of coffee will give you get-up-and-go, make you feel awake and alert, but so will amphetamines— and caffeine is in the same class of drugs. And because it's legal, accessible, and socially acceptable, it's rarely thought of as addictive or dangerous—but it is both!

Caffeine is a *drug*. It's in coffee, tea, colas, chocolate, and numerous medications, and can cause dependency and adverse reactions that most people are not aware of.

WHY CAFFEINE'S UNFIT FOR ANY FORM OF FITNESS:
- It can induce anxiety, headaches, irritability, nervousness, and insomnia.
- It can increase palpitations and heart irregularities.
- It can raise blood pressure.
- It can cause adverse digestive and bowel problems in sensitive individuals.
- Excessive intake of methylxanthines—or xanthines— (active chemicals in caffeine) can cause benign breast disease and prostate problems.
- It can interfere with DNA replication.

- The amount contained in about 4 cups of coffee daily could cause birth defects.
- It depletes the body of such needed nutrients as vitamin B_1, inositol, biotin, potassium, zinc, and can also inhibit calcium and iron assimilation.

JUDGE HOW MUCH CAFFEINE YOU'RE GETTING

BEVERAGE OR FOOD	MG. CAFFEINE
Roasted or ground coffee (8 oz. cup)	85–150
Instant coffee (8 oz. cup)	60
Decaffeinated coffee (8 oz. cup)	15
Tea (8 oz. cup)	40–120
Cocoa (8 oz. cup)	6–42
Cola beverages (12 oz.)	35–70
Chocolate (1 oz.)	6

POPULAR DRUGS THAT HIDE 100 OR MORE MILLIGRAMS OF CAFFEINE:
- Cafergot Tablets
- Migralam Capsules
- Bio Slim T Capsules
- Dexatrim
- Dietac Capsules
- Nodoz
- Prolamine
- Slim One Capsules
- Vivarin

YOUR BEST NUTRITIONAL DEFENSE

- MVP (see section 38)
- Vitamin B complex, 100 mg., 1–3 times daily

- L-tryptophan (500–667 mg.), 1–3 times daily with water, no protein
- Chelated calcium and magnesium, 3 tabs, 3 times daily

131. Recreational, Illicit, and Abused Drugs: The Higher You Get, the Harder You Fail

AMPHETAMINES

Often used for an easy emotional up, amphetamines stimulate the central nervous system and produce adrenalinelike effects that cause your heart, blood, and pulse pressure to rise, getting all your bodily systems going at high speed, creating feelings of increased ability, alertness, and euphoria.

Unfortunately, when the drug begins to wear off (anywhere between four and fourteen hours), nervousness, paranoia, and fatigue set in, along with headache and palpitations. Most users find that the only remedy for this syndrome (known as "crashing") is to take more amphetamine. And since tolerance develops quickly, more and more of the drug is needed to produce the original effect.

SERIOUS SECOND THOUGHTS FOR USERS:
- One large dose or repeated small doses over an extended period of time can cause amphetamine psychosis (a toxic reaction), which can last from several days to several weeks.
- Heavy users can develop tremors or malnutrition, and increase their susceptibility to disease and infection.
- Memory loss and delusions may exist up to a year after the drug is discontinued.

SHAPE-UP NUTRITION

- Niacinamide and vitamin C, 1,000 mg. each, taken 3 times daily after meals. (Can restore energy levels and alleviate discomforts of the comedown.)
- A high-potency multiple vitamin with chelated minerals, 1–3 times daily; calcium-rich diet (see section 36); and plenty of liquids. (Can help users get back on a healthy, drug-free track.)

COCAINE

Another central-nervous-system stimulant that produces a feeling of fast-and-easy emotion energy, intense self-confidence, and a loss of appetite. But these effects are short-lived (about one half hour), and more coke is needed to recapture the high.

Nasal inhalation is the most popular form of taking the drug, but it's also often applied under the eyelids and tongue (because it's absorbed rapidly through mucous membranes); it can be injected intravenously, or smoked in a process called "free basing." Though not physically addictive, psychological dependence is high.

SERIOUS SECOND THOUGHTS FOR USERS:

- Repeated use of large amounts can cause nosebleeding, the feeling that bugs are crawling on or under your skin, cold sweats, nausea, vomiting, increased heartbeat and body temperature, convulsions, and anaphylactic shock.
- Toxicity is unpredictable because even small doses with the wrong cut can be dangerous for sensitive individuals.
- Cocaine poisoning, caused by too rapid absorption of

the drug—usually through intravenous injection—can result in immediate death.

SHAPE-UP NUTRITION

- High-potency multiple vitamin and mineral, A.M. and P.M.
- High-potency chelated multiple mineral, A.M. and P.M.
- Vitamin C, 1,000 mg., 1–3 times daily (essential for repairing abused nasal tissues)
- Vitamin E (dry form), 200–400 IU, 1–3 times daily
- Vitamin B complex, 100 mg., 1–3 times daily (an important stress fighter, and needed to replace lost B vitamins)

- *And to kick the habit:* Tyrosine, mixed in orange juice, and tyrosine hydroxylase (the enzyme that lets the body use tyrosine) along with supplements listed above. (Cocaine addicts at Fair Oaks Hospital in Summit, New Jersey, used this regimen for 12 days and the results were remarkably effective, especially in alleviating the depression, fatigue, and irritability that make quitting so difficult.)

MARIJUANA AND HASHISH

Though the chemical and psychological effects of these drugs vary with individuals, they essentially act as relaxants, tranquilizers, appetite-stimulants, intoxicants, enhancers of the senses, and mild hallucinogens.

Unlike most other illicit and recreational drugs, marijuana and hashish have the curious property of "reverse tolerance," which means that seasoned users need *less* of the drug to get high than first-timers. This is most likely caused by tetrahydrocannabinol (THC)—the psychoactive ingredient in marijuana and hash—accumulating in the body, requiring only a small additional amount for a regular user to achieve an effect.

SERIOUS SECOND THOUGHTS FOR USERS:

- Unwarranted panic can occur (usually in users who have had little or no prior drug experience).
- A preexisting depressed mood can be intensified.
- If cannabis is eaten and the amount ingested has been underestimated, toxic psychosis can result.
- Anyone with a preexisting mental disorder runs the risk of a psychotic reaction.
- Smoking marijuana raises blood pressure and can increase the risk of lung cancer; smoking marijuana during pregnancy can cause low birth weight in newborns.

SHAPE-UP NUTRITION

- MVP (see section 38)
- Extra vitamin C, 1,000 mg. (time release), A.M. and P.M.
- Vitamin B complex, 100 mg., 1–3 times daily. (Those "munchies" you've gotten have probably provided you with more than your share of B-thieving sugars and carbohydrates.)
- Vitamin E (dry form), 200–400 IU, 1–3 times daily (to protect your lungs)

132. Smoking Won't Help Your Nerves— Or Any Other Part of You

The reason most smokers feel that puffing on a cigarette "helps" their nerves is essentially because nicotine provides a stimulus barrier that protects the brain from unpleasant or distracting external stimuli, such as annoying noises, arguments, or distressing situations of any kind.

But whatever emotion-easing benefits you might think you're deriving from smoking, the risks to your total health and well-being far outweigh them.

WHY YOU SHOULD PUT THAT CIGARETTE OUT OF YOUR LIFE

Cigarette smoking can . . .

- cause cancer of the lung, larynx, mouth, esophagus, bladder, kidney, and pancreas;
- cause chronic bronchitis and emphysema;
- interact adversely with oral contraceptives to increase the probability of coronary and cerebrovascular disease;
- increase the risk of spontaneous abortion and prenatal death;
- cause coronary heart disease;
- retard fetal growth, lower birth weight of infants, impair growth and development during early childhood;
- worsen symptoms of respiratory and cardiovascular disease;
- deplete the body of vitamin C;
- change the way many drugs are metabolized in the body;
- increase the risk of lung cancer among nonsmokers exposed to cigarette smoke;
- elevate blood pressure;
- and much more!

HIGHLY RECOMMENDED SUPPLEMENTS

(The following regimen is no substitute for quitting, but it can give your body a fighting chance for health.)

- High-potency multiple vitamin with chelated minerals (time release), A.M. and P.M. (with meals)
- High-potency chelated multiple mineral, A.M. and P.M. (with meals)
- Vitamin C, 1,500–3,000 mg., daily
- Vitamin E (dry form), 400–1,000 IU, daily
- Selenium, 50 mcg., 1–3 times, daily
- Vitamin A, 10,000 IU, daily for 5 days, then stop for 2
- Cysteine, 500–1,000 mg., daily

133. Why It's So Tough To Quit

Aside from nicotine being physically addictive, it gets smokers used to having a buffer against certain distressing external stimuli. When you quit smoking, your brain no longer has this buffer, and suddenly stimuli of all sorts come charging at you with an unpleasant reality that's greater than if you'd never smoked at all—hence, withdrawal symptoms.

GOOD NEWS FOR BREAKING THE HABIT

Smokers can now break their habit—without having to give up nicotine at the same time. A nicotine chewing gum (Nicorette) is available at pharmacies (though a prescription is required). Each piece contains approximately 2–4 mg. of nicotine, and one package of gum is said to be the nicotine equivalent of a pack of twenty cigarettes.

SUPPLEMENTS FOR AN EASIER WITHDRAWAL

- L-tryptophan (500–667 mg.), 3 times daily, between meals, with water
- Vitamin B complex, 100 mg., 1–3 times daily
- Vitamin C, 1,500 mg., 1–3 times daily
- High-potency vitamin with chelated minerals, A.M. and P.M.
- Chelated Zinc, 15–50 mg., 1–3 times daily

134. Any Questions About Chapter VII?

My mother takes Inderal, a heart medication, and for the past several months has been depressed. I've asked her doctor if the pill was depleting her of some necessary vitamins, and he said her blood tests showed no deficiencies. I still feel that there's some connection between her medication and her moods. Her doctor is willing to prescribe an antidepressant, but I'd rather he didn't. As a pharmacist, and a nutritionist, what's your opinion?

My opinion is that you're very perceptive. There are a lot of drugs that people don't realize could cause depression, but can—and beta-blockers, such as Inderal, are among them. Others include Lioresal (baclofen), Darvon (propoxyphene), Tigan (trimethobenzamide), adrenocorticoids, antihypertensives, estrogens, antiarthritis medicines, potassium supplements, *procainamide*, and any sort of sex hormones. Before rushing out for a prescription for your mother, I'd suggest trying to increase her intake of emotion-upping foods (see section 122), as well as a vitamin B complex, 100 mg., 3 times daily; vitamin C, 1,000 mg., 1–3 times daily; calcium and magnesium, 3 tabs, 3 times daily; and L-tryptophan, 500–667 mg., 1–3 times daily.

I was told that a bath before bedtime would relax me and help me sleep. How come that every time I take one, I feel wide awake?

Possibly because the water is too *hot*. Hot water will wake you up. *Warm* water is what you want. That's what soothes and relaxes muscles. Sip a cup of chamomile tea in the tub, pat yourself dry when you get out, and you'll probably be off to dreamland before you can count that second sheep. (See section 78 for supplements that can help.)

I'm not a regular drinker, but when I do go out on the weekend and have a few, I always wind up with a hangover that really hangs me up for the whole next day. Are there any supplements that would help?

You'll be happy to know that there are. Before going out, take 100 mg. of a vitamin B complex. During that evening (if you can remember to do it), take another one, and still another before going to bed.

If you forget to do this, or still awake with a hangover, the following regimen should shape you up:

- Vitamin B_1, 1,000 mg.
- Cysteine, 500 mg.
- Vitamin B_{12}, 100 mcg.
- Vitamin C, 1,500 mg.

Even though I'm a carpet salesman, I'm known in my family as "the absentminded professor." This is probably a long shot, but are there any vitamins that can improve memory?

It's not a long shot at all. There are indeed memory-enhancing supplements. I'd advise the following:

- Choline, 1–5 g., daily, in divided doses
- L-glutamine, 500 mg., 3 times daily
- Vitamin B complex, 50–100 mg., 1–3 times daily
- RNA-DNA, 300 mg. daily (CAUTION: Do not take if you have gout, as this can increase serum uric acid levels)
- *Tyrosine, 500–2,000 mg., daily (taken at bedtime or upon waking, with water—no protein)
- *Phenylalanine, 500–2,000 mg., daily (taken at bedtime or upon waking, with water—no protein)
- Vitamin C, 1,000 mg., 1–3 times daily

*CAUTION: Tyrosine and phenylalanine are contraindicated in certain types of skin cancer. They should not be taken with MAO inhibitors—or other drugs, without checking with a doctor—because they can elevate blood pressure; they are not recommended for use during pregnancy, and should not be taken by anyone with PKU (phenylketonurea).

TIME OUT

There's Nothing Fake About Psychosomatic Illness

The word *psychosomatic*, Greek in origin, means "mind-body." It does not mean "caused by the mind."...This is a gross misunderstanding, because the whole point of the word psychosomatic is that the mind and body are both involved. Neither does psychosomatic mean *hypochondriacal*. Hypochondria is the tendency to imagine that you are sick when you are not. Psychosomatic illnesses are real.

Dr. Andrew Weil, author of
*Health and Healing: Understanding
Conventional and Alternative Medicine*

Think about it...

VIII.

Sexual Fitness

135. Sex: Nature's Most Revitalizing Exercise

Probably the most enjoyable physical, emotional, and energy-renewing "aerobic" workout is sex.

* It tones the heart, lungs, and entire cardiovascular system.
* It can relax and energize the body.
* It can elevate hormone levels, particularly in women, which increases muscular strength and vitality.
* Regular sexual activity can help the body produce hormones capable of aiding the body in retaining such important energizing minerals as potassium, sodium, sulfur, chloride, and phosphorus.
* Twenty minutes of active sex can burn up as many as 200 calories.
* A drop in sexual activity, according to Dr. Thomas P. Hackett of the American Heart Association, often precedes heart attacks, while a resumption of nonstressful satisfactory sex seems to be a key to progress in rehabilitation following heart attacks.

136. Sensual Nutrients, Herbs, and Potions

THINK ZINC TO HIGH-POWER YOUR SEX DRIVE: A deficiency in zinc can cause a definite deficit in your sex drive. To get your love life back into high gear, increase your intake of foods such as oysters, wheat germ, wheat bran, pumpkin seeds, meat, and seafood, and supplement with 50 mg. of chelated zinc, 1–3 times daily.

THE SEXUAL STIMULANT THAT'S BEEN AROUND——FOR CENTURIES: Ginseng, often called "manroot" because of its resemblance to the human body, has been used around the world for centuries as a sexual stimulant. Slices of the root can be chewed, or prepared as a tea or tonic. (It's also available in tablet form.) Because ginseng has a normalizing effect on the body's metabolism, it reduces stress, which is an asset when it comes to increasing sexual pleasure.

VITAMIN E COULD MEAN ECSTASY: Vitamin E increases fertility in males and females and aids in the proper function of all nerves and muscles. That it directly influences the sex drive has yet to be conclusively proven, but I have met many happy vitamin-E zealots who are convinced that it does. A diet high in wheat germ, vegetable oils, soybeans, eggs, and whole-grain cereals, along with a daily supplement of 200–400 IU dry form vitamin E, 1–3 times daily, could mean the difference between a night of passion . . . and, well, just a night.

AN UNCOMPLEX SEX PROBLEM SOLUTION——WITH VITAMIN B COMPLEX: Though vitamin B complex is not directly an aphrodisiac, it is a definite stress reducer, and coupled with zinc, it has been found to help cure numerous cases of impotence. Eat plenty of wheat germ, fish, melon, and cabbage—and supplement with 50–100 mg. of vitamin B complex, 1–3 times daily.

DAMIANA—AN HERB THAT SERVES PASSION BY THE CUP: Damiana, an herb also known as turnea, has long been touted as a natural aphrodisiac. It's easily made into a tea by pouring a cup of boiling water over a teaspoonful of the dried leaves or one-quarter teaspoonful of the ground leaf powder. For best results, have you or your partner drink one to four cups daily.

SARSAPARILLA—WORLD-CLASS APHRODISIAC: Sarsaparilla is probably one of the most widely known—and used—aphrodisiacal herbs. As a tea it has been used as a successful sexual stimulant through the centuries by the Indians of Mexico. (The sarsaparilla plant has chemical substances with testosterone, progesterone, and cortisol activity, which may account for the plant's usefulness in increasing sexuality.) Well-satisfied users recommend boiling one ounce of this root in a pint of water for half an hour and drinking wine-size glassfuls frequently.

And if you're looking for a love potion, the following has been alleged to be the tastiest and best:

Cupid's Midnight Special

½ cup banana (pureed)

½ cup watermelon juice

1 cup papaya juice

1 tsp. ground cloves

Blend and sip slowly.

137. Rx's That Can Nix Your Sex Life

Some of the most widely used medications can adversely affect the sexual desire as well as sexual performance of both men and women. Individuals with a history of sexual problems are most susceptible to these sorts of side effects, but they *can* happen to anyone.

SEX-SABOTAGING MEDICINES

The drugs listed below may cause any or all of the following: decreased sexual desire, delayed orgasm, ejaculation difficulties, impotence.

DRUG	TYPE
Amitriptyline (Elavil)	Antidepressant
Baclofen (Lioresal)	Muscle relaxant
Benztropine (Cogentin)	Anticholinergic
Chlordiazepoxide (Librium)	Tranquilizer/sedative
Chlorphentermine (Pre-Sate) *(Causes problems primarily in women.)*	Amphetamine
Chlorthalidone (Hygroton)	Diuretic
Chlorotrianisene (Tace) *(Causes problems in men only.)*	Hormone
Cimetidine (Tagamet) *(Can also lower sperm count.)*	Ulcer medication

DRUG	TYPE
Clofibrate (Atromid-S)	Cholesterol reducer/ antihyperlipemic
Clonidine (Catapres)	Antihypertensive
Cyclobenzaprine (Flexeril)	Muscle relaxant
Desipramine (Norpramin)	Antidepressant
Dextroamphetamine (Amodex, Benzedrine) *(Causes problems primarily in women.)*	Amphetamine
Diazepam (Valium)	Tranquilizer/sedative
Dienestrol (Dienestrol Cream) *(Causes problems in men only.)*	Hormone
Diethylpropion (Tenuate, Tepanil) *(Causes problems primarily in women.)*	Amphetamine
Diphenhydramine (Benadryl, etc.)	Antihistamine
Disopyramide (Norpace)	Antiarrhythmic
Esterfied estrogens (Estratab, Evex, Menrium) *(Causes problems in men only.)*	Hormone
Estradiol (Estrace) *(Causes problems in men only.)*	Hormone

DRUG	TYPE
Estrone (Menagen) *(Causes problems in men only.)*	Hormone
Ethionamide (Trecator)	Antituberculosis
Fenfluramine (Pondimin) *(Causes problems primarily in women.)*	Amphetamine
Guanethidine (Ismelin) *(Causes decreased emission of semen.)*	Antihypertensive
Hydralazine (Apresoline, etc.)	Antihypertensive
Hydrochlorothiazide (Hydrodiuril)	Diuretic
Hydroxyzine (Vistaril, Atarax)	Tranquilizer
Imipramine (Tofranil)	Antidepressant
Isocarboxazid (Marplan)	Antidepressant
Isopropamide (Darbid)	Antispasmodic
Levodopa (Dopar, etc.)	Antidyskinetic
Lithium (Lithonate, Lithane)	Antidepressant
MAO Inhibitors *(Women may lose ability to achieve orgasm while retaining sexual desire.)*	Antidepressant

DRUG	**TYPE**
Meprobamate (Equanil, Miltown)	Tranquilizer/sedative
Methantheline (Banthine)	Antispasmodic
Methyldopa (Aldomet)	Antihypertensive
Metoprolol (Lopressor)	Antihypertensive
Norethindrone (Norlutin)	Hormone
Norgestrel (Ovrette)	Hormone
Orphenadrine (Norflex, etc.)	Muscle relaxant
Oxazepam (Serax)	Tranquilizer/sedative
Pargyline (Eutonyl)	Antidepressant
Perhexilene (Pexid)	Antianginal
Phenelzine (Nardil)	Antidepressant
Phenoxybenzamine (Dibenzyline)	Antihypertensive
Progesterone (Progestasert, Progestin)	Hormone
Propantheline (Pro-banthine)	Antispasmodic
Propanolol (Inderal, Inderide)	Antihypertensive

DRUG	TYPE
Protriptyline (Vivactil)	Antidepressant
Reserpine (Demi-regroton, Diupres, Ser-Ap-Es, Serpasil)	Antihypertensive
Spironolactone (Aldactone)	Diuretic
Thioridazine (Mellaril) *(Causes ejaculatory difficulties without impairing orgasm.)*	Tranquilizer
Tranylcypromine (Parnate)	Antidepressant
Trihexyphenidyl (Artane)	Anticholinergic

138. Accelerating Your Sex Drive with Supplements

* Phenylalanine, 250–500 mg., daily
* Tyrosine, 250–500 mg., daily
* Vitamin C, 1,000 mg., 1–3 times daily
* Vitamin A, 5,000–10,000 IU, daily 5 days a week (stop for 2)
* Vitamin E (dry form), 400–800 IU, daily
* Chelated zinc, 15–50 mg., daily
* Selenium, 50–100 mcg., daily
* Vitamin B complex, 50 mg., 1–3 times daily

OPTIONAL: Siberian ginseng tea (or capsules), 3 times daily

For men only: Pumpkin seed oil (vitamin F), 3 capsules daily

For postmenopausal women only: Mixed tocopherol vitamin E, 400 IU, daily

139. Solving Prostate Problems Without Surgery

The prostate gland is universally accepted as the governor of male sexual health. It normally contains about ten times more zinc than any other organ in the body, but when there is benign hypertropy (enlargement) of the prostate, scientists have found that zinc concentrations are lower than normal. In chronic prostatitis (where there is often infection as well as enlargement), the zinc concentration is even lower. In cancerous prostate conditions, zinc levels are lowest of all.

Treating prostate sufferers with zinc-rich diets and supplements has shown to be remarkably effective. In many cases, symptoms have disappeared completely. I'd suggest increasing your intake of brewer's yeast, wheat bran, oysters, onions, rice, eggs, and lentils, among other high-zinc foods. (See section 36.)

A SUPPLEMENT REGIMEN

- MVP (see section 38)
- Chelated zinc, 50 mg., 3 times daily
- Vitamin F or lecithin capsules (1,200 mg.), 3 caps, 3 times daily

140. Shaping Up After Vasectomy

Vasectomy is a relatively simple, safe, sterilization procedure where the vas deferens (the male's sperm-carrying tubes) are sealed, preventing the ejaculation of sperm. The sperm continue to be formed, but are resorbed into body tissues.

Because of this, many antibodies are engaged in continually inactivating sperm, often causing a man who has had a vasectomy to become more susceptible to infections.

Since most men have vasectomies in order to continue an active sex life, it's wise to take out nutritional insurance to ensure it.

RECOMMENDED NUTRITIONAL INSURANCE

- MVP (see section 38)
- Extra vitamin C, 1,000 mg., A.M. and P.M.
- Chelated zinc, 15–50 mg., daily

141. VD and Vitamin Demands

SYPHILIS

Syphilis is caused by a tiny corkscrewlike organism called a spirochete. It is usually transmitted by sexual contact and requires only the presence of an open wound or slightly irritated mucous membrane, such as the mouth, rectum, or outer male and female genital organs, to enter the body.

In its first stage, there is usually a painless sore on the penis or entrance to the vagina. (The sore might appear instead, or also, on the nipple, anus, or finger.)

In its second stage (one to two months later), there

is a mild general illness, sore throat, mild fever, and a pink nonitchy rash. (Third stage symptoms, which can endanger virtually all organs, appear four or more years later, but are extremely rare, as the disease is usually diagnosed by then.)

If early treatment is started with penicillin or any of the other newer antibiotics, recovery is swift and complete. Unfortunately, some of these remedies cause almost as much need for supplements as the disease itself. (See regimen below.)

GONORRHEA

Like syphilis, gonorrhea is usually transmitted through sexual contact, but the responsible organism, the gonococcus, has the ability to acquire a resistance to some of the most powerful medical weapons, such as sulfa drugs, penicillin, and many of the -mycins.

Symptoms occur three to ten days after infection. There is usually pain on passing urine and a discharge of pus. Often these symptoms go unnoticed by women.

Early and adequate treatment with antibiotics is essential in order to avoid complications. But, as I've mentioned before, though these remedies do their job, they take their nutritional toll out on you.

RECOMMENDED SUPPLEMENT

- MVP (see section 38)
- Extra vitamin C, 1,000 mg., A.M. and P.M.
- (3 acidophilus capsules, 3 times daily; and vitamin K, 100 mcg., daily, if on an extended antibiotic program.)

142. Dietary Help for Genital Herpes

WHAT IS GENITAL HERPES?

Genital herpes (herpes simplex II) is a painful rash located on the skin or inner membranes of the vagina, penis, or anus. It is caused by a virus, and is transmitted mainly through sexual contact. The infection, when first contracted, may be accompanied by a high fever, even meningitis.

Symptoms usually disappear in about two weeks, but, ironically, the virus does not. Instead, it remains latent until some other event (infection, fever, emotional stress, fatigue) reactivates it and causes it to travel down the nerve fibers to again produce pain and rash at the original site.

Once you have a primary herpes infection, it may occur repeatedly, recur a few times and then stop, or simply lie dormant in the body nerve tissues and not produce symptoms for a lifetime. But there's always the chance that it can be reactivated by stress, and it's more than likely to be reactivated upon physical contact with another person with active genital herpes.

FOODS THAT CAN FIGHT BACK

Although not conclusively tested against placebos (inactive substances used to compare test results), there is mounting evidence that large dietary intakes of the amino acid lysine—and extremely minimal intakes of the amino acid arginine (see section 36)—can be an effective preventive as well as therapy for herpes infections.

LOAD UP ON LYSINE:
DAIRY PRODUCTS

Cottage cheese (uncreamed)—1 cup	3,584 mg.
Egg—1 med.	400 mg.
Milk, skim, dry, instant—1 cup	1,780 mg.

FISH

Flounder, baked—1 lb.	11,880 mg.
Salmon, pink, canned—1 lb.	8,081 mg.
Shrimp, cooked—1 lb.	7,225 mg.
Tuna, canned, drained—1 lb.	11,504 mg.

FRUITS

Fig, raw—1 med.	117 mg.
Avocado	240 mg.
Strawberries—1 cup	48 mg.

MEATS, POULTRY

Liver, fried—1 lb.	6,772 mg.
Beef, rump roast—1 lb.	8,526 mg.
Lamb—1 lb.	9,543 mg.
Ham, roasted—1 lb.	7,807 mg.

NUTS AND SEEDS

Almonds, dried—1 cup	774 mg.
Peanuts, roasted, with skin—1 cup	2,592 mg.
Pumpkin and squash kernels—1 cup	3,068 mg.

VEGETABLES

Green beans—1 cup	104 mg.
Bean sprouts (mung)—1 cup	218 mg.
Cauliflower, raw—1 cup	151 mg.
Chick-peas (garbanzos), dry raw—½ cup	1,415 mg.
Green peas (cooked)—1 cup	338 mg.
Soybeans, cooked—1 cup	1,518 mg.

BREAD
Pumpernickel—1 slice   119 mg.

FLOUR
Soy—1 cup   2,784 mg.

143. Any Questions About Chapter VIII?

*I am a 35-year-old woman, in good physical health,
sexually active, but have difficulty achieving orgasm. I've
gone the therapy route, and it didn't work. Are there any
nutritional, drug, or other solutions to my problem?*

I'd suggest you look over the list of sex-elevating
vitamins and herbs mentioned in section 136; make sure
by checking with your doctor or pharmacist that you're
not taking any medication that could interfere with your
sex life (also check listing in section 137); and try "Kegeling"
—an exercise that has helped numerous women with
your problem.

Kegeling is simply a tightening and releasing of the
vaginal muscles. (To be sure that you're doing it correctly,
start by practicing to stop and start your urine flow.)
These are the same muscles that are involved in sexual
intercourse, and shaping them up can only help.

Additionally, you might want to try a potion developed
by Ursula Le Cordier, author of *The High Sexuality Diet*
(Arrow Publications). Put a peeled cucumber, a pint of
natural yogurt, and a dash of pepper in the blender and
mix until frothy. Garnish with a sprinkle of cinnamon.
Even if it doesn't help you sexually, it will nutritionally.

Is it true that cocaine is an aphrodisiac?

Quite the contrary. And it's an expensive and dangerous disappointment for those who think so. In fact,
the more you use, the less able you are to perform

sexually. Though it might prolong intercourse for some, it reduces sensation and usually inhibits orgasm. That's not what I'd call an aphrodisiac.

Do you know of any exercises for men that could improve sexual fitness?

The ones I've found are almost all Oriental, designed to integrate body and mind—much like yoga and t'ai chi. This is not to say that they are in any way ineffective—in fact, they're quite the opposite. But they're not as simple as sit-ups and do require concentrated effort and practice.

There is a book called *TSFR: The Taoist Way to Total Sexual Fitness for Men* by Bruce M. Wong (Golden Dragon Publishers, Princeton, NJ: 1982), which gives explicit, step-by-step exercises, and would probably be worth your looking into. In the meanwhile, any good aerobic exercise, combined with proper rest and nutrition, and a supplement of 15–50 mg. chelated zinc, daily, will help promote your general fitness—which includes sex.

TIME OUT

Exercise Versus Valium

People who exercise say that the world takes on a
rosier glow. . . . We believe that neurohormones
in the brain are altered by physical activity; that
may alter your mood, and improve your coping
skills. After exercise the muscles are as relaxed as
they are after a dose of tranquilizing medication.
It's likely that untensed muscles are a good indication of an untensed psyche, too.

Dr. John Farquhar, Director
Stanford Heart Disease Prevention Program
Stanford University Medical School

Think about it . . .

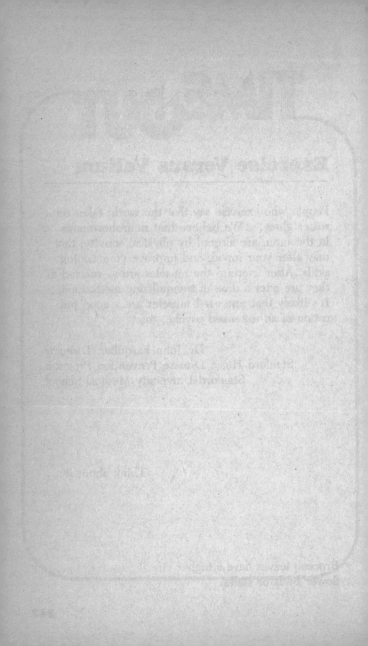

IX.

Finish Line

144. How To Get Maximum Nutrition from Your Food

- Make salads when you're ready to eat them. Cut-up fruits and vegetables that are left to stand lose vitamins.
- Wash but don't soak fresh vegetables; soaking can diminish important B and C vitamins.
- Cut or shred fresh vegetables with a sharp knife because vitamins A and C are reduced when vegetable tissues are bruised.
- To get more calcium, iron, and vitamin A from your lettuce, use the coarser outer green leaves, which have a higher concentration of these nutrients than the inner leaves.
- Buy flash-frozen fruits or vegetables if you're not planning to eat them right away. The vitamin content of good frozen green beans will be higher than those fresh ones you've kept in the refrigerator for a week.
- Don't thaw frozen vegetables before cooking.
- Broccoli leaves have a higher vitamin A value than the flower buds or stalks.

- Converted and parboiled rice has more vitamins than polished rice, and brown rice is more nutritious than white.
- Frozen foods that can be boiled in their bags provide more vitamins than the ordinary kind; and all frozen foods are preferable to canned ones.
- Cooking in copper pots (not pots with copper bottoms) can destroy vitamin C, folic acid, and vitamin E.
- Stainless steel, glass, and enamel are the best utensils for retaining nutrients while cooking. (Iron pots can give you the benefit of that mineral but will shortchange you on vitamin C.)
- The shorter the cooking time and the less water used will give you the most nutrients.
- Keep milk that is in glass containers out of the light to prevent loss of riboflavin and vitamins A and D. (Breads exposed to light can also lose these nutrients.)
- For extra nutrition, use cooking water from vegetables for making soups, juices from meats for gravies, and syrups from canned fruits to make desserts.
- Well-browned, crusty, or toasted baked goods have less thiamine than others.
- Boil or bake potatoes in their skins to get the most nutrients from them.
- You lose the thiamine and vitamin C benefits of vegetables if you use baking soda while cooking them.
- Store fruits and vegetables in the refrigerator as soon as you bring them home.

145. How To Locate a Nutritionally Oriented Doctor

For a list of nutritionally oriented practitioners in your area, write to the following organizations. Be sure to enclose a stamped, self-addressed envelope.

International College of Applied Nutrition
Box 386
La Habra, CA 90631

International Academy of Preventative Medicine
10950 Grandview, Suite 469
Overland Park, KS 66210

International Academy of Metabiology, Inc.
P.O. Box 15157
Las Cruces, NM 88001

Prevention Magazine Readers' Service
Emmaus, PA 18049

Consulting Nutritionists in Private Practice
P.O. Box 345
Cold Springs, NY 10515

American Academy of Medical Preventics
8383 Wilshire Blvd., Suite 922
Beverly Hills, CA 90211

American Holistic Medical Association
6932 Little River Turnpike
Annandale, VA 22003

The Huxley Institute
219 East 31 Street
New York, NY 10016
(distributes information on both orthomolecular psychiatry and medicine)

Northwest Academy of Preventive Medicine
15615 Bellevue-Redmont Road, Suite E
Bellevue, WA 98008

146. Free Calls for Health Help

For information about venereal or sexually transmitted diseases (STD), you can call Operation Venus: 1-800-272-2577

For the latest health news from the American Medical Association, you can call: 1-800-621-8094

For information about cancer, the National Cancer Institute will answer any question they can. Just call: 1-800-4-CANCER

For information about Alzheimer's disease, the National Alzheimer's Disease Foundation can help. Call: 1-800-621-0379

147. Write-away for Fitness

(Enclose a stamped, self-addressed envelope with all queries.)

Bicycling	Bikecentennial—The Bicycle Travel Association P.O. Box 8308 Missoula, MT 59807
Hiking and backpacking	Sierra Club 530 Bush Street San Francisco, CA 94108
Jogging and running	American Running and Fitness Association 2420 K Street NW Washington, DC 20037
Swimming	International Amateur Swimming Foundation 200 Financial Center Des Moines, IA 50309

Walking   Walking Association
                               4113 Lee Highway
                               Arlington, VA 22207

148. Any Questions About Chapter IX?

What agency would be best to contact for information about understanding government regulations and the food industry?

Send a stamped, self-addressed envelope with your query to: Center for Science in the Public Interest, 1755 S Street NW, Washington, DC 20009.

Are there any organizations to help concerned citizens find out the safety of their local food supply?

Yes. For help I'd advise you contact: Federation of Homemakers, P.O. Box 5571, Arlington, VA 22205. Send a stamped, self-addressed envelope with your query.

Is there any organization that can help insomniacs?

For a list of sleep disorder clinics around the country, send a stamped, self-addressed envelope with your query to: Association for Sleep Disorders Center (ASDC), Box 2604, Del Mar, CA 92014.

What's the address of Alcoholics Anonymous?

They're usually listed in your local telephone directory, but you can write to the national office: Alcoholics Anonymous, P.O. Box 459, Grand Central Station, New York, NY 10163.

Afterword

I sincerely hope that I have given you a greater understanding of fitness and how important it is— on all levels—to your health and happiness. Even more, I hope I've been able to provide enough practical information on body, mind, drug, and nutrition connections not only to encourage but also to enable you to achieve and maximize whatever individual health and happiness goals you seek.

I have always believed that people could be all that they wanted to be if they had enough desire and guidance. My aim, therefore, has been to fuel that desire and supply guidance as well.

This book was written to be consulted, as one would a knowledgeable friend, and has been intrinsically committed to personal enlightenment on a flexible day-to-day basis, with leeway always allowed for growth and change. By condensing essentials and simplifying technicalities, pinpointing specifics and indicating further areas of study, I fondly wish that all of you will be able to find a way, for yourself and for your loved ones, to enjoy the fruits of fitness for life.

EARL L. MINDELL, R.Ph., Ph.D.

Beverly Hills, California
October 1984

Glossary

Absorption: The process by which nutrients are passed into the bloodstream.

Acetate: A derivative of acetic acid.

Acetic acid: Used as a synthetic flavoring agent, one of the first food additives (vinegar is approximately 4 to 6 percent acetic acid); it is found naturally in cheese, coffee, grapes, peaches, raspberries, and strawberries. Generally Recognized As Safe (GRAS) when used only in packaging.

Acetone: A colorless solvent for fat, oils, and waxes, which is obtained by fermentation (inhalation can irritate lungs, and large amounts have a narcotic effect).

Acid: A water-soluble substance with sour taste.

Addiction: Compulsive use of habit-forming drugs.

Adrenal gland: A triangular-shaped gland near each kidney that synthesizes and stores dopamine, norepinephrine, and epinephrine.

Adrenals: The glands, located above each kidney, that manufacture adrenaline.

Alkali: An acid-neutralizing substance (sodium bicarbonate is an alkali used for excess acidity in foods).

Allergen: A substance that causes an allergy.

Allergy: Abnormal sensitivity to any substance.

Amenorrhea: Absence or suppression of menstruation.

Amino acid chelates: Chelated minerals that have been produced by many of the same processes nature uses to chelate minerals in the body; in the digestive tract, nature surrounds the elemental minerals with amino acid, permitting them to be absorbed into the bloodstream.

Amino acids: The organic compounds from which proteins are constructed; there are twenty-two known amino acids, but only nine are indispensable nutrients for men—histidine, isoleucine, leucine, lysine, total S-containing amino acids, total aromatic amino acids, threonine, tryptophan, and valine.

Amnesia: Memory loss.

Anabolic: A building up of body substance; a constructive phase of metabolism; a conversion of nonliving material into living cytoplasm of cells.

Analgesic: Drug used to relieve pain.

Anemia: Reduction in normal amount of red blood cells.

Aneurysm: Localized abnormal dilation of a blood vessel; may be due to congenital defect or weakness of blood vessel wall.

Angina pectoris: Severe attacks of pain about the heart, caused by an insufficient supply of blood to the heart.

Anorectic: Having no appetite.

Anorexia: Loss of appetite.

Anorexia nervosa: A symptom of mental disturbance that causes loss of appetite for food and compulsive dieting.

Antibiotic: Any of various substances that are effective in inhibiting or destroying bacteria.

Anticholinergic: See **antispasmodic.**

Anticoagulant: Something that delays or prevents blood clotting; blood-thinner.

Antidyskinetics: Drugs used in the treatment of Parkinson's disease.

Antiemetic: Remedy to prevent vomiting.

Antigen: Any substance not normally present in the body that stimulates the body to produce antibodies.

Antihistamine: A drug used to reduce effects associated with colds and allergies.

Antineoplastics: Drugs that prevent growth and development of malignant cells.

Antioxidant: A substance that can protect another substance from oxidation; added to foods to keep oxygen from changing the food's color.

Antispasmodic: A drug used to relieve cramping and spasms of the stomach, intestines, and bladder.

Antitoxin: An antibody formed in response to—and capable of—neutralizing a poison of biologic origin.

APC: Aspirin (acetylsalicylic acid), phenacetin, and caffeine; common combination of ingredients in a variety of cold remedies and analgesics.

Aphrodisiac: An agent that produces sexual desire.

Apnea: Temporary cessation of breathing, usually during sleep.

Arthritis: Inflammation of joints.

Aspirin: Acetylsalicylic acid, used to relieve headaches, pain, fever, and inflammation.

Assimilation: The process whereby nutrients are used by the body and changed into living tissue.

Asthma: Condition of lungs characterized by decrease in diameter of some air passages; a spasm of the bronchial tubes or swelling of their mucous membranes.

Ataxia: Loss of coordinated movement.

ATP: A molecule called adenosine triphosphate, the fuel of life, a nucleotide—building block of nucleic acid—

that produces biological energy with B_1, B_2, B_3, and pantothenic acid.

Avidin: A protein in egg white capable of inactivating biotin.

Bariatrician: A weight-control doctor.

Beta-adrenergic blocking agent: A substance that blocks the transmission of stimuli thereby slowing down the rate of nerve response in the heart, and the heart rhythm itself.

"Beta-blocker": See **beta-adrenergic blocking agent.**

BHA: Butylated hydroxyanisole; a preservative and antioxidant used in many products; insoluble in water; can be toxic to the kidneys.

BHT: Butylated hydroxytoluene; a solid, white crystalline antioxidant used to retard spoilage of many foods; can be more toxic to the kidney than its nearly identical chemical cousin BHA.

Bioflavonoids: Usually from orange and lemon rinds, these citrus-flavored compounds needed to maintain healthy blood-vessel walls are widely available in plants, citrus fruits, and rose hips; known as vitamin P-complex.

Bradycardia: Slow heart rate.

Calciferol: A colorless, odorless crystalline material, insoluble in water; soluble in fats; a synthetic form of vitamin D made by irradiating ergosterol with ultraviolet light.

Calcium gluconate: An organic form of calcium.

Capillary: A minute blood vessel, one of many that connect the arteries and veins.

Carcinogen: A cancer-causing substance.

Cardiac arrhythmia: Irregular heart action caused by disturbances in discharge of cardiac impulses.

Cardiovascular: Pertaining to heart and blood vessels.

Carotene: An orange-yellow pigment occurring in many

plants and capable of being converted into vitamin A in the body.

Casein: The protein in milk that has become the standard by which protein quality is measured.

Catabolism: The metabolic change of nutrients or complex substances into simpler compounds, accompanied by a release of energy.

Catalyst: A substance that modifies, especially increases, the rate of chemical reaction without being consumed or changed in the process.

Cataract: Clouding of the lens of the eye, which prevents clear vision.

Catecholamines: Epinephrine and norepinephrine; biologically active amines derived from the amino acid tyrosine; produce marked effects on the nervous and cardiovascular systems, metabolic rate, temperature, and smooth muscle.

Cellulose: A fibrous nondigestible carbohydrate; aids in intestinal elimination; provides no nutrient value.

Chelation: A process by which mineral substances are changed into easily digestible form.

Chronic: Of long duration; continuing; constant.

Cirrhosis: A chronic liver disease characterized by dense or hardened connective tissue, degenerative changes or alteration in structure.

CNS: Central nervous system.

Coenzyme: The major portion, though nonprotein, part of an enzyme; usually a B vitamin.

Cold sores: Lesions, particularly in and around the mouth, caused by herpes simplex virus.

Colitis: Inflammation of large intestine.

Collagen: The primary organic constituent of bone, cartilage, and connective tissue (becomes gelatin through boiling).

Coma: Complete loss of consciousness.

Congenital: Condition existing at birth, not hereditary.

Corticosteroid: Any of various steroid substances obtained from the adrenal gland.

Corticosterone: An adrenal cortex hormone that influences the metabolism of carbohydrates, potassium, and sodium; essential for normal absorption of glucose.

Cortisone: An adrenal gland hormone; also used as an anti-inflammatory agent.

Dehydration: A condition resulting from an excessive loss of water from the body.

Dermatitis: An inflammation of the skin; a rash.

Desiccated: Dried; preserved by removing moisture.

Dicalcium phosphate: A filler used in pills that is derived from purified mineral rocks and is an excellent source of calcium and phosphorus.

Diluents: Fillers; inert material added to tablets to increase their bulk in order to make them a practical size for compression.

Diuretic: Increases flow of urine from the body.

DNA: Deoxyribonucleic acid; the nucleic acid in chromosomes that is part of the chemical basis for hereditary characteristics.

Dopamine: A compound that increases blood pressure.

Dysmenorrhea: Painful or difficult menstruation.

Dyspepsia: Indigestion.

Edema: Excessive accumulation of tissue fluid.

Endogenous: Produced from within the body.

Enteric coated: A tablet coated so that it dissolves in the intestine, not in the stomach (which is acid).

Enteritis: Inflammation of the intestines, particularly the small intestines.

Enzyme: A protein substance found in living cells that brings about chemical changes; necessary for digestion of food.

Epidermis: The outer layer of skin.

Epilepsy: Convulsive disorder.

Epinephrine: Produced by the adrenal medulla and other tissues, it has also been synthesized and is used as a vasoconstrictor, heart stimulant, and to relieve asthmatic attacks.

Estrogens: Female sex hormones.

Excipient: Any inert substance used as a dilutant or vehicle for a drug.

Exogenous: Derived or developed from external causes.

FDA: Food and Drug Administration.

Fibrin: An insoluble protein that forms the necessary fibrous network in the coagulation of blood.

Free radicals: Highly reactive chemical fragments that can produce an irritation of artery walls, start the arteriosclerotic process if vitamin E is not present; generally harmful.

Fructose: A natural sugar occurring in fruits and honey; called fruit sugar; often used as a preservative for foodstuffs and an intravenous nutrient.

Gallstones: Stonelike objects found in gall bladder and its drainage system.

Glaucoma: Disease of the eyes in which the pressure of the fluid in the eye increases.

Glucose: Blood sugar; a product of the body's assimilation of carbohydrates and a major source of energy.

Glutamic acid: An amino acid present in all complete proteins; usually manufactured from vegetable protein; used as a salt substitute and a flavor-intensifying agent.

Glutamine: An amino acid that constitutes, with glucose, the major nourishment used by the nervous system.

Gluten: A mixture of two proteins—gliadin and glutenin—present in wheat, rye, oats, and barley.

Glycogen: The body's chief storage carbohydrate, primarily in the liver.

Gout: Upset in metabolism of uric acid, causing inflammation of joints, particularly in the knee or foot.

GRAS: Generally Recognized As Safe; a list established by Congress to cover substances added to food.

Half-life: The time it takes for half the amount of a drug to be metabolized or inactivated (disappear from the bloodstream) by the body (an important consideration for determining the amount and frequency of drug dosage).

Hallucination: False perception having no relation to reality and not accounted for by any exterior stimuli; may involve one, all, or any combination of the senses.

Hepatitis: Inflammation of liver.

Hesperidin: Part of the C-complex.

Holistic treatment: Treatment of the whole person.

Homeostasis: The body's physiological equilibrium.

Hormone: A substance formed in endocrine organs and transported by body fluids to activate other specifically receptive organs.

Humectant: A substance that is used to preserve the moisture content of materials.

Hydrochloric acid: A normally acidic part of the body's gastric juice.

Hydrolyzed: Put into water-soluble form.

Hydrolyzed protein chelate: Water-soluble and chelated for easy assimilation.

Hypertension: High blood pressure.

Hypervitaminosis: A condition caused by an excessive ingestion of vitamins.

Hypoglycemia: Low blood sugar.

Hypotension: Low blood pressure.

Hypovitaminosis: A deficiency disease owing to an absence of vitamins in the diet.

Ichthyosis: A condition characterized by a scaliness on the outer layer of skin.

Idiopathic: Describes a condition whose causes are not yet known.

Immune: Protected against disease.

Infectious: Liable to be transmitted by infection.

Inflammation: Changes that occur in living tissues when invaded by germs; swelling, pain, heat.

Insulin: The hormone, secreted by the pancreas, concerned with the metabolism of sugar in the body.

IU: International Units.

Jaundice: Increase in bile pigment in blood, causing yellow tinge to skin, membranes, and eyes; can be caused by disease of liver, gallbladder, bile system, or blood.

Lactating: Producing milk.

Lactation: Secretion of milk by breasts.

Laxative: A substance that stimulates evacuation of the bowels.

Linoleic acid: One of the polyunsaturated fats, a constituent of lecithin; known as vitamin F; indispensable for life, and must be obtained from foods.

Lipid: A fat or fatty substance.

Lipofuscin: Age pigment in cells.

Lipotropic: Preventing abnormal or excessive accumulation of fat in the liver.

MAO Inhibitors: Abbreviation for monoamine oxidase inhibitors; a group of antidepressants that promotes an elevation of levels of amine messengers in the emotional regions of the brain.

Megavitamin therapy: Treatment of illness with massive amounts of vitamins.

Menopause: Age at which normal cessation of monthly period occurs, usually between 45 and 50.

Metabolize: To undergo change by physical and chemical processes.

Mitochondria: The powerhouse of energy in the cell; they are involved in protein synthesis and lipid metabolism.

Narcotic: A central nervous system depressant which, in moderate doses, relieves pain and produces sleep; in large doses it can produce unconsciousness or even death; can be addicting.

Nausea: Stomach discomfort with the feeling of a need to vomit.

Neuron: Nerve cell.

Neurotransmitter: A chemical that transports messages between neurons in the brain.

Nitrites: Used as fixatives in cured meats; can combine with natural stomach and food chemicals to cause dangerous cancer-causing agents called nitrosamines.

Norepinephrine: A hormone produced by the adrenal medulla, similar to epinephrine, and used chiefly as a vasoconstrictor.

Obesity: Excessive stoutness.

Ophthalmia: Inflammation of eye.

Ophthalmic: Pertaining to eyes.

Orthomolecular: The right molecule used for the right treatment; doctors who practice preventive medicine and use vitamin therapies are known as orthomolecular physicians.

OSHA: Occupational Safety and Health Administration.

Osteoporosis: A condition characterized by porous (softening or increasingly brittle) bones.

Oxalates: Organic chemicals found in certain foods, especially spinach, which can combine with calcium to form calcium oxalate, an insoluble chemical the body cannot use.

PABA: Para-aminobenzoic acid; a member of the B-complex.

Palmitate: Water-solubilized vitamin A.

Parasite: Any animal or plant that lives inside or on the body of another animal or plant.

Peptic: Pertaining to digestive tract.

Photosensitivity: Sensitivity to light.

PKU (phenylketonuria): A hereditary disease caused by the lack of an enzyme needed to convert an essential amino acid (phenylalanine) into a form usable by the body; can cause mental retardation unless detected early.

Polyunsaturated fats: Highly nonsaturated fats from vegetable sources; tend to lower blood cholesterol.

Poultice: A soft, moist mass of herbs, oils, medicine, etc., spread on a cloth and applied to the skin to relieve congestion or pain.

Predigested protein: Protein that has been processed for fast assimilation and can go directly to the bloodstream.

Provitamin: A vitamin precursor; a chemical substance necessary to produce a vitamin.

Psoriasis: A skin condition characterized by silver-scaled red patches.

Psychosis: Type of insanity in which one loses almost complete touch with reality.

PUFA: Polyunsaturated fatty acid.

RDA: Recommended Dietary Allowances as established by the Food and Nutrition Board, National Academy of Sciences, National Research Council.

Rhinitis: Inflammation of the lining of the nose.

RNA: Ribonucleic acid.

Rose hips: A rich source of vitamin C; the nodule underneath the bud of a rose called a hip, in which the plant produces the vitamin C we extract.

Rutin: A substance extracted from buckwheat; part of the C-complex.

Saturated fatty acids: Usually solid at room temperature; higher proportions found in foods from animal sources; tend to raise blood cholesterol levels.

Sequestrant: A substance that absorbs ions and prevents changes that would affect flavor, texture, and color of food; used for water softening.

Soporific: Producing sleep.

Steroid hormones: The sex hormones and hormones of the adrenal cortex.

Steroids: A family of cortisonelike medications; prescribed when adrenal glands do not produce enough of the hormone cortisone; also used for treatment of swellings, allergic reactions, and other conditions.

Sulfonamides: A group of sulfa drugs used to treat specific infections that are not responsive to other antibacterials.

Synergistic: The action of two or more substances to produce an effect that neither alone could accomplish.

Synthetic: Produced artificially.

Systemic: Pertaining to the whole body.

Tachycardia: Rapid beating of heart coming on in sudden attacks.

Teratogen: Anything that causes the development of abnormalities in an embryo.

Tocopherols: The group of compounds (alpha, beta, delta, epsilon, eta, gamma, and zeta) that make vitamin E; obtained through vacuum distillation of edible vegetable oils.

Topical: Applied externally.

Toxicity: The quality or condition of being poisonous, harmful, or destructive.

Toxin: An organic poison produced in living or dead organisms.

Tremor: Shake or quiver.

Triglycerides: Fatty substances in the blood.

Ulcer: Sore or lesion on skin surface or internal mucous membranes.

Unsaturated fatty acids: Most often liquid at room temperature; primarily found in vegetable fats.

Urticaria: Skin eruptions that are associated with severe itching; hives.

USAN: United States Adopted Names Council; cosponsored by the American Pharmaceutical Association

(APhA), the American Medical Association (AMA), and the United States Pharmacopia (USP) for the specific purpose of coining suitable, acceptable, nonproprietary names in the drug field.

USRDA: United States Recommended Daily Allowances.

Vasodilator: A drug that dilates (widens) blood vessels.

Xerosis: A condition of dryness.

Zein: Protein from corn.

Zyme: A fermenting substance.

Bibliography and Recommended Reading

I am greatly indebted to a vast number of nutritionists, pharmacists, doctors, scientists, therapists, fitness counselors, researchers, government agencies, and authors whose works in the fields of nutrition, fitness, pharmacology, and medicine not only inspired, but enabled me to complete a long-desired project that would otherwise have been impossible.

The list that follows is given to show my sincere and wholehearted appreciation. Many of the books are highly technical, but others, which have been marked with an asterisk, I would like to recommend to all concerned individuals for further reading in areas of your own particular interest or specialized nutrition and fitness needs.

*Abrahamson, E. M., and Pezet, A. W. Body, Mind and Sugar. New York: Avon Books, 1977.
*Adams, Ruth. The Complete Home Guide to All the Vitamins. New York: Larchmont Books, 1972.
*Adams, Ruth, and Murray, Frank. Minerals: Kill or Cure. New York: Larchmont Books, 1976.

*Airola, Paavo. *Hypoglycemia, A Better Approach*. Phoenix, AZ: Health Plus, 1977.

*Bailey, Hubert. *Vitamin E: Your Key to a Healthy Heart*. New York: ARC Books, 1964, 1966.

*Bennett, William, and Gurin, Joel. *The Dieter's Dilemma*. New York: Basic Books, 1982.

*Berkow, Robert, ed. *The Merck Manual*. 14th ed. Rahway, NJ: Merck and Co., 1982.

Bieri, John G. "Fat-soluble vitamins in the eighth revision of the Recommended Dietary Allowances." *Journal of the American Dietetic Association* 64 (February 1974).

Billups, Norman F. *American Drug Index 1982*. Philadelphia: J. B. Lippincott, 1982.

*Blau, Sheldon Paul, and Schultz, Dodi. *Arthritis*. New York: Doubleday, 1973.

*Borsaak, Henry. *Vitamins: What They Are and How They Can Benefit You*. New York: Pyramid Books, 1971.

*Brace, Edward R. *The Pediatric Guide to Drugs and Vitamins*. New York: Dell, 1982.

*Bricklin, Mark. *Practical Encyclopedia of Natural Healing*. Emmaus, PA: Rodale Press, 1976.

*Breithaupt, Sandra, and Agnew, Wayne. *The Dallas Doctors Diet*. New York: McGraw-Hill, 1983.

*Brody, Jane. *The New York Times Guide to Personal Health*. New York: Times Books, 1982.

*Burack, Richard, with Fox, Fred J. *New Handbook of Prescription Drugs*. Rev. New York: Ballantine Books, 1980.

*Burns, David D. *Feeling Good, The New Mood Therapy*. New York: New American Library, 1980.

Burton, Benjamin. *Human Nutrition*. 3rd ed. New York: McGraw-Hill, 1976.

*Cammer, Leonard. *Up From Depression*. New York: Pocket Books, 1969.

*Clark, Linda. *Know Your Nutrition*. New Canaan, CT: Keats Publishing, 1973.

*————. *Secrets of Health and Beauty*. New York: Jove Publications, 1977.

Consumer Reports 40. "Marijuana: The Health Questions." March 1975.

Consumer Reports. "How Nutritious Are Fast Food Meals?" May 1975.

Consumer Reports 43. "Too Much Sugar." March 1978.

Consumer Reports, Editors of. *The Medicine Show*. Mount Vernon, NY: Consumers Union, 1981.

*Cooper, Kenneth. *Aerobics*. New York: Bantam Books, 1968.

Cumulative Index for Journal of Applied Nutrition. La Habra, CA: International College of Applied Nutrition, 1947–76, 1976.

*de Bairacli Levy, Juliette. *Common Herbs for Natural Health*. New York: Schocken Books, 1974.

Deckert, Robert. "Ant Bites Relieve Arthritis." *Omni*, February 1983.

*DiCyan, Erwin, and Hessman, Lawrence. *Without Prescription*. New York: Simon & Schuster, 1972.

*Dominguez, Richard H. *Total Body Training*. New York: Warner Books, 1983.

The Drug Abuse Survey Project. *Dealing with Drug Abuse*. A Report to the Ford Foundation. New York: Praeger, 1972.

*Dufty, William. *Sugar Blues*. Philadelphia: Chilton Book, 1975.

*Ebon, Martin. *Which Vitamins Do You Need?* New York: Bantam Books, 1974.

*Edelstein, Barbara. *The Woman Doctor's Diet for Women*. New York: Prentice-Hall, 1977.

*Evens, Wayne O., and Cole, Jonathan O. *Your Medicine Chest*. Boston: Little, Brown & Co., 1978.

Flynn, Margaret A. "The Cholesterol Controversy." *Journal of the American Pharmacy*, NS18 (May 1978).

"Food Facts Talk Back." *Journal of the American Dietetic Association*, 1977.

*Frank, Benjamin S. *No-Aging Diet*. New York: Dial, 1976.

*Fredericks, Carlton. *Eating Right for You*. New York: Grosset and Dunlap, 1972.

*_____. *Look Younger/Feel Healthier*. New York: Grosset and Dunlap, 1977.

*_____. *Psycho Nutrients*. New York: Grosset and Dunlap, 1976.

*Freudenberger, Herbert J. *Burnout: The High Cost of High Achievement*. New York: Anchor Press, 1980.

*Gomez, Joan, and Gerch, Marvin J. *Dictionary of Symptoms*. New York: Bantam Books, 1972.

Goodhart, Robert S., and Shills, Maurice E. *Modern Nutrition in Health and Disease*. 5th ed. Philadelphia: Lea and Febiger, 1973.

*Gottlieb, Annie, and Sher, Barbara. *Wishcraft: How To Get What You Really Want*. New York: Ballantine, 1983.

*Graedon, Joe. *The People's Pharmacy*. New York: St. Martin's Press, 1976.

_____. *The People's Pharmacy*. Vol. 2. New York: Avon Books, 1980.

*Gutin, Bernard, with Kessler, Gail. *The High-Energy Factor*. New York: Random House, 1983.

*Haas, Robert. *Eat To Win: The Sports Nutrition Bible*. New York: Rawson Associates, 1984.

*Haimes, Leonard, and Tyson, Richard. *How To Triple Your Energy*. New York: New American Library, 1978.

Harper, Alfred E. "Recommended Dietary Allowances: Are They What We Think They Are?" *Journal of the American Dietetic Association* 64 (February 1974).

Howe, Phyllis S. *Basic Nutrition in Health and Disease*. 6th ed. Philadelphia: W. B. Saunders, 1976.

International College of Applied Nutrition. *Nutrition—Applied Personally*. La Habra, CA, 1978.

Journal of the American Dietetic Association. "Vitamin-Mineral Safety, Toxicity, and Misuse." 1978.

Katz, Marcella. *Vitamins, Food, and Your Health*. Public Affairs Committee, 1971, 1975.

Krupp, M. A., and Chatton, M. J. *Current Medical Diagnosis and Treatment*. Los Altos: Long Medical Publications, 1982.

*Kurtz, Irma. *Beds of Nails and Roses: A Guide to Your Emotions*. New York: Dodd, Mead, 1983.

LaPlace, John. *Health*. New York: Appleton-Century-Crofts, 1972.

*Levy, Stephan J. *Managing Drugs in Your Life*. New York: McGraw-Hill, 1983.

*Linde, Shirley. *The Whole Health Catalog*. New York: Rawson Associates, 1977.

*Lucas, Richard. *Nature's Medicines*. New York: Prentice-Hall, 1966.

*Lust, John. *The Herb Book*. New York: Bantam Books, 1974.

*Madders, Jane. *Stress and Relaxation*. New York: Arco, 1979.

*Martin, Alice A., and Tenenbaum, Frances. *Diet Against Disease*. Boston: Houghton Mifflin, 1980.

*Martin, Clement G. *Low Blood Sugar: The Hidden Menace of Hypoglycemia*. New York: Arco, 1976.

Martin, Marvin. *Great Vitamin Mystery*. Rosemont, IL: National Dairy Council, 1978.

*Mason, David, and Dyller, Fran. *Pharmaceutical Dictionary and Reference for Prescription Drugs*. New York: Playboy Paperbacks, 1981.

*Mayer, Jean. *A Diet for Living*. New York: David McKay, 1975.

Medical Economics. *Physician's Desk Reference*. 36th ed. Oradell, NJ: Medical Economics Co., 1982.

Mitchell, Helen S. "Recommended Dietary Allowances Up To Date." *Journal of the American Dietetic Association* 64 (February 1974).

National Dairy Council. *Nutrition Source Book*. Rosemont, IL: 1978.

National Health Federation Bulletin, November 1978.

National Nutrition Consortium, American Dietetic Association. *Nutrition Labeling: How It Can Work For You*. 1975.

National Nutrition Education Clearing House. *Nutrition Information Resources for the Whole Family*. 1978.

National Research Council. *Recommended Dietary Allowances*. 8th ed., rev. Washington, DC: National Academy of Sciences, 1974.

————. *Toxicants Occurring Naturally in Foods*. 2nd ed. Washington, DC: National Academy of Sciences, 1973.

*Newbold, H. L. *Dr. Newbold's Revolutionary New Discovery about Weight Loss*. New York: Rawson Associates, 1977.

*————. *Mega-Nutrients for Your Nerves*. New York: Peter H. Wyden, 1978.

New York State Medical Society Drug Abuse Committee. *Desk Reference on Drug Misuse and Abuse*. New York, 1981.

*Null, Gary and Steve. *The Complete Book of Nutrition*. New York: Dell, 1972.

Nutrition Almanac. New York: McGraw-Hill, 1979.

Nutrition Foundation. *Index of Nutrition Education Materials*. Washington, DC: 1977.

Nutrition Foundation. "Present Knowledge in Nutrition." *Nutrition Reviews*, 1976.

*Panos, Maesimund, and Heimlich, Jane. *Homeopathic*

Medicine at Home. Los Angeles: J. P. Tarcher, 1980. Distributed by Houghton Mifflin, Boston.

*Passwater, Richard A. *Super Nutrition*. New York: Dial, 1975.

*Pauling, Linus. *Vitamin C and the Common Cold*. New York: Bantam Books, 1971.

*Pearson, Durk, and Shaw, Sandy. *Good News for Smokers*. Huntington Beach, CA: The International Institute of Natural Health Sciences, 1980.

*_____. *Life Extension*. New York: Warner Books, 1982.

*Phillips, Joel L., and Wynne, Ronald D. *Cocaine: The Mystique and the Reality*. New York: Avon Books, 1980.

*Poe, William D. *The Old Person in Your Home*. New York: Scribner's, 1969.

*Pomeranz, Virginia E., and Schultz, Dodi. *The Mothers' and Fathers' Medical Encyclopedia*. New York: New American Library, 1977.

*Pritikin, Nathan. *The Pritikin Permanent Weight-Loss Manual*. New York: Grosset and Dunlap, 1981.

*Rodale, J. I. *The Complete Book of Minerals for Health*. 4th ed. Emmaus, PA: Rodale Books, 1976.

*_____ *The Encyclopedia of Common Diseases*. Emmaus, PA: Rodale Press, 1976.

Roe, Daphne A. *Handbook: Interactions of Selected Drugs and Nutrients in Patients*. Chicago: The American Dietetic Association, 1982.

*Rosenberg, Harold, and Feldzaman, A. N. *Doctor's Book of Vitamin Therapy: Megavitamins for Health*. New York: Putnam, 1974.

*Rubinstein, Morton K. *A Doctor's Guide to Non-Prescription Drugs*. New York: New American Library, 1977.

*Ruthe, Eshleman, and Winston, Mary, comps. *The American Heart Association Cookbook*. New York: Ballantine, 1973.

*Saffon, M. J. *Body Lifts*. New York: Warner Books, 1984.

*Samuels, Mike, and Bennett, Hal. *The Well Body Book*. New York: Random House, 1973.

*Seaman, Barbara and Gideon. *Women and the Crisis in Sex Hormones*. New York: Rawson Associates, 1977.

*Sehnert, Keith W., with Eisenberg, Howard. *How To Be Your Own Doctor*. New York: Grosset and Dunlap, 1975.

*Shute, Wilfrid E., and Taub, Harold J. *Vitamin E for Ailing and Healthy Hearts*. New York: Pyramid Books, 1969.

*Silverman, Harold M., and Simon, Gilbert I. *The Pill Book*. 2nd ed. New York: Bantam Books, 1982.

*Spock, Benjamin. *Baby and Child Care*. New York: Simon & Schuster, 1976.

Thomas, Clayton I., ed. *Tabers Cyclopedia Medical Dictionary*. 13th ed. Philadelphia: F. A. Davis, 1977.

Underwood, Eric J. *Trace Elements in Human and Animal Nutrition*. 4th ed. New York: Academic Press, 1977.

United Nations. Food and Agriculture Organization. *Calorie Requirements*, 1957, 1972.

U.S. Department of Agriculture. *Amino Acid Content of Food*, by M. L. Orr and B. K. Watt; 1957; rev. 1968.

U.S. Department of Agriculture, Consumer and Food Economics Institute, Agricultural Research Service. *Composition of Foods: Raw, Processed, Prepared*, by Bernice K. Watt and Annabel L. Merrill, 1975.

U.S. Department of Agriculture. *Energy Value of Foods: Basis and Derivation*, by Annabel L. Merrill and Bernice K. Watt, 1973.

U.S. Department of Agriculture. *Nutritive Value of American Foods*, by Catherine F. Adams, 1975.

U.S. Department of Health, Education and Welfare. *Consumer Health Education: A Directory*, 1975.

The United States Pharmacopeial Convention. *The Physicians' and Pharmacists' Guide to Your Medicines*. New York: Ballantine, 1981.

U.S. President's Council on Physical Fitness and Sports. *Exercise and Weight Control*, by Robert E. Johnson. Urbana, IL: University of Illinois Press, 1967.

U.S. Senate Select Committee on Nutrition and Human Needs. *Diet and Killer Diseases with Press Reaction and Additional Information*. Washington, DC: U.S. Government Printing Office, 1977.

U.S. Senate Select Committee on Nutrition and Human Needs. *National Nutrition Policy: Nutrition and the Consumer II*. Washington, DC: U.S. Government Printing Office, 1974.

*Wade, Carlson. *Health Tonics, Elixirs and Potions for the Look and Feel of Youth*. West Nyack, NY: Parker Publishing, 1971.

*_____. *Magic Minerals*. West Nyack, NY: Parker Publishing, 1967.

*_____. *Miracle Protein*. West Nyack, NY: Parker Publishing, 1975.

*_____. *Vitamin E: The Rejuvenation Vitamin*. New York: Award Books, 1970.

*Weil, Andrew. *Health and Healing: Understanding Conventional and Alternative Medicine*. Boston: Houghton Mifflin, 1983.

Williams, Roger J. *Nutrition Against Disease*. New York: Pitman Publishers, 1971.

*Winter, Ruth. *A Consumer's Dictionary of Food Additives*. New York: Crown, 1978.

*Wolfe, Sidney M., and Coley, Christopher M. *Pills That Don't Work*. New York: Farrar, Straus & Giroux, 1980.

*Yanker, Gary D. *The Complete Book of Exercise Walking*. New York: Contemporary Books, 1983.

*Young, Klein, Beyer. *Recreational Drugs*. New York: Berkley, 1982.

*Yudkin, John. *Sweet and Dangerous*. New York: Peter H. Wyden, 1972.

Index

A

Acetominophen, 38, 40
Achilles tendon, stretching, 47
Acidophilus, skin and, 143
Acne, 149–150
Activity. *See* Exercise
Adrenal gland concentrates.
    See Glandulars
Aerobic dancing, 17
Aerobic exercise, 15–19
    cytochrome C and, 8–9
    joints and, 47
    sex as, 229
    skin and, 144
    walking and, 29
After-shave lotions, 151–152
Age
    arthritis and, 183
    determination of target
        heart zone and, 20–22
    need for stress test and, 13
    nutrition during pregnancy
        in over thirty mothers

and, 124–126
    swimming stroke selection
        and 30–31
    See also Older persons
Aging, immune system and,
    201
Air pollution, 47
Alcohol intake
    emotional health and, 213–
        214
    exercise and, 48
    nutrients decreasing desire
        for, 214–215
    during pregnancy, 137–138
    skin damage and, 145
    supplements for hangovers
        from, 224
    Vitamin B-complex and, 7
    zinc and, 4
Alcoholics Anonymous, 251
Alfalfa, during pregnancy, 126
Allergies
    to aspirin, 38
    care of, 189–190

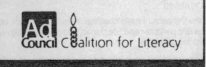